BIOETHICS
AND
SOCIAL REALITY

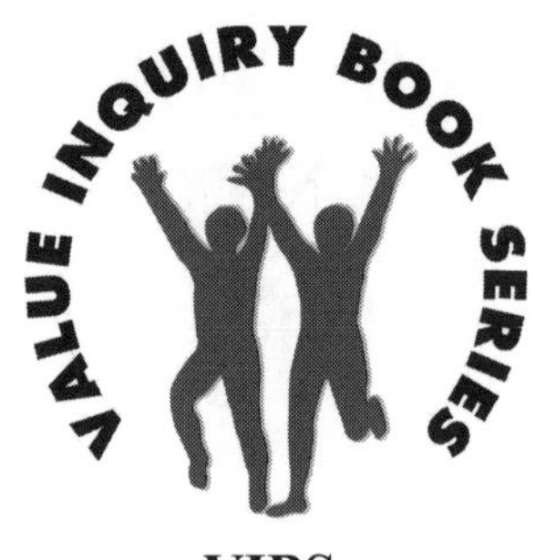

VIBS

Volume 165

a volume in
Values in Bioethics
ViB
Matti Häyry and Tuija Takala, Editors

BIOETHICS
AND
SOCIAL REALITY

Matti Häyry, Tuija Takala,
and Peter Herissone-Kelly, Editors

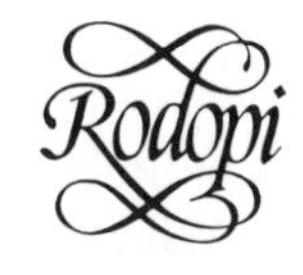

Amsterdam - New York, NY 2005

Cover Design: Studio Pollmann

The paper on which this book is printed meets the requirements of "ISO 9706:1994, Information and documentation - Paper for documents - Requirements for permanence".

ISBN: 90-420-1655-8

Printed in the Netherlands

CONTENTS

FOREWORD

This second book to come from bioethicists working in the North West of England demonstrates not only the power, strength, and depth of the talent available here, but is also very much a tribute to a strong gale of fresh Nordic air. The initiative—and indeed the energy required to bring that initiative to fruition—has very much come from our North-Easterly neighbors in Denmark and Finland: Matti Häyry, Tuija Takala, and Søren Holm. Although Søren has now moved a little South of us to what might be called the Central West, he will remain an honorary Mancunian. The editors of this volume are right to say that we have not only in this and the preceding volume the beginnings of an institution in terms of publication, but also that we very clearly have, here in the North West, a major bioethics institution in European terms. Taken as a whole, the North West group of bioethicists and medical lawyers can reasonably claim to constitute both the largest and the most active centre for bioethics in Europe.

The present volume addresses the social reality of bioethics. No topic could be more pressing and important at this time. Many of the most crucial questions that face humanity are related to the life sciences and the way in which those sciences may be used and abused by humankind. Not only the social reality that faces us today, but the social reality that will face our descendents, depends upon how we use the scientific and technological tools that have been and are being developed. Indeed, how we use these tools will determine whether our descendents—both in the near and the far future—remain human beings, properly so called, or become some new breed of persons that we will, in part, have created. Many current writers look with horror and distaste upon the prospect of changing the fundamental nature of humanity. In recent times Francis Fukuyama and Leon Kass have both made eloquent appeals for the preservation of our species. Others, including Jonathan Glover, myself, and Gregory Stock, have taken a more pragmatic approach to the desirability of what will be an increasingly artificial preservation of this particular species. We know that not only all human beings that now exist but all primates, gorillas, chimpanzees, gibbons, orangutans, and siamangs are descended from a common ape ancestor who lived in Africa between 5,000,000 and 7,000,000 years ago. If our common ancestor had had the foresight or the power to take the view that has been taken by Fukuyama or Kass, we would never have existed to debate the issue of the preservation of humankind. As Richard Dawkins has elegantly pointed out recently, we humans are not only apes, we are African apes, and this is a natural category which does not permit the artificial separation out of human beings.

It is difficult to imagine a more important topic for study than that of the social reality of bioethics, the reality within which it exists, and which it will help to shape in the future. How we manage that reality will determine not only the nature of our lives and the shape of our societies, but indeed our very identity as self-conscious beings.

The essays in this volume are all stimulating, important, and original contributions to bioethics. I have much enjoyed and appreciated the opportunity this book has given me to think again about the issues they raise, and to engage with the stimulating, provocative, and sometimes frightening insights that they contain.

Professor John Harris
Sir David Alliance Professor of Bioethics
University of Manchester
May 2004

PREFACE

This book marks the birth of a very special series. Following *Scratching the Surface of Bioethics*, edited by Matti Häyry and Tuija Takala (VIBS 144), it is the second volume produced by a group of bioethicists in the North West of England, at the universities of Central Lancashire, Keele, and Manchester. One book does not make a series—but two might just indicate the beginnings of an institution.

Most chapters in this book are based on presentations given in the Second North West Bioethics Roundtable (NorthWeb 2), organized by Professor Søren Holm in Manchester on 3 February 2003. Some additional thematically-related papers were solicited from scholars who could not attend the meeting, but whose work complements the original contributions.

The sponsors of NorthWeb 2, and the ensuing book project, included

- *Empirical Methods in Bioethics*, a project co-ordinated by Professor Søren Holm and funded by the European Union Quality of Life and Management of Living Resources research program;
- *Genes, Information, and Business*, a project co-ordinated by Professor Matti Häyry and funded by the Academy of Finland research program Life 2000;
- *Ethical and Social Aspects of Bioinformatics*, a project co-ordinated by Professor Matti Häyry and funded by the Academy of Finland research program Systems Biology and Bioinformatics;
- *What Is Bioethics All About?* a project co-ordinated by Dr Tuija Takala and funded by the Helsingin Sanomain 100 Years Foundation;
- *Values in Bioethics*, a Special Series in Rodopi's *Value Inquiry Book Series*;
- *Centre for Social Ethics and Policy*, University of Manchester;
- *Institute of Medicine, Law, and Bioethics*, University of Manchester;
- *Centre for Professional Ethics*, University of Central Lancashire; and
- *Faculty of Health*, University of Central Lancashire.

The organizers, and the editors of this book, acknowledge this support with gratitude. In addition, the editors would like to thank Tony Quinn and Peter Neill for invaluable help with recalcitrant computers.

Matti Häyry, Tuija Takala, Peter Herissone-Kelly
18 April 2004, Manchester and Preston, England

Introduction

THE SOCIAL REALITY OF BIOETHICS

Matti Häyry, Tuija Takala, and Peter Herissone-Kelly

1. What Is Social Reality?

The title of this book presented some initial problems to many of our authors. "What is 'social reality?'" they asked. Should we not rather be talking about the different meanings or interpretations that can be given to reality? And is there a "reality," as opposed to these various readings?

The definition of "social reality" in the following chapters is wide. It includes all the spheres of human interaction which we call social and which somehow exist in conjunction with the physical, material, cultural, and moral worlds we inhabit. It includes all the fields of human activity that Georg Wilhelm Friedrich Hegel referred to as "civil society"—education, work, commerce, and voluntary associations—but also aspects of family life and social policy that he classified in different categories.[1] Medicine, health-care, and scientific advances in biology and genetics, too, are in many ways intertwined with these realms.

Bioethics as an activity is, of course, also an increasingly important part of social reality, widely construed. Professional self-regulation, legislation, and ethical studies have an impact on education and social policy, and also on the other manifestations of our lives together. Social reality and bioethics exist in a reciprocal relationship, where changes in one frequently reflect or cause changes in the other.

2. Classical Concerns

In the first three chapters of the book, three philosophers address some of the classical concerns in bioethics, namely those evoked by sex, death, and drugs. In the contexts of abortion, suicide, and cannabis prescriptions, they discuss the degree to which consequences, duties, and personal autonomy should be taken into account in laws and regulations.

In chapter one, Harry Lesser examines the case of back-street abortion—the argument that terminations of pregnancy should be legally allowed, because their prohibition inflicts serious harm on women who have to, and will, resort to the services offered by incompetent and dangerous abortionists. According to his analysis, those who believe that abortions are morally wrong cannot be conceptually forced to accept the argument, since the consequences in this particular case are too difficult to assess and interpret. He argues, however, that in more straightforward cases, ineffective laws which can be seen to have harmful effects should not be implemented, and if they have already been implemented, they ought to be repealed. He also argues that although empirical facts do not always determine legal issues, they should still be discovered and taken into account.

In chapter two, Doris Schroeder scrutinizes the possibility of physician-assisted self-sacrifice in the face of medical scarcity. She distinguishes between three main categories: namely, physician-assisted self-sacrifice, altruistic physician-assisted suicide, and obligatory honorable physician-assisted suicide. These are all theoretically feasible, but her argument is that while the first two can in certain circumstances be legitimate, the third option is always immoral, since it violates the requirement of respect for the autonomy of individuals. The element of coercion present in honorable suicides implies a culturally determined duty to die, which cannot be justified. The risk of coercion is also an element in the other two classes, which is why vulnerable groups should not be encouraged to sacrifice themselves for the sake of others.

In chapter three, Matti Häyry studies the use of the concepts of autonomy and freedom in relation to cannabis prescriptions for pain management. He maintains that autonomy, or self-determination, as the notion is currently understood in bioethics, would probably support restrictions on the use of cannabis for medicinal purposes. The restrictions are based on the idea that drugs like this confuse the mind and lead to addiction—both presumably factors that would hinder rational and moral decision making. He argues, however, that different normative conclusions would be reached by employing the idea of freedom as non-restriction of options, and defends the view that freedom instead of autonomy should be respected in situations where individuals are not harming others by decisions which render them less than autonomous in the demanding moral sense.

3. Developments

The next three chapters deal with developments in medical technology and the relevance of popular claims, attitudes, and evaluations. The authors take on questions related to the assignment of parenthood in surrogacy disputes, arguments for and against human reproductive cloning, and the relevance of feelings of disgust in the context of new medical technologies.

In chapter four, Monique Jonas analyzes the competing claims of genetic and surrogate parents for primary care-taking responsibility for the children they jointly produce. She identifies three bases for such claims: the genetic connection between biological parents and their children, labor put into the childbearing process, and contracts made concerning the surrogacy arrangement. She argues that since genetics and labor can produce equally noteworthy consequentialist arguments for the competing sides in the usual type of dispute, claims founded on surrogacy contracts should be used to break the tie. According to her, only women who are reasonably sure that they will not change their minds during the pregnancy ought to enter into such contracts. If they do change their minds, they should not be blamed in any way, but the original agreement should, nonetheless, be honored.

In chapter five, Tuija Takala explores the rights and wrongs of human reproductive cloning. The objections that she considers include the arguments from dignity, uniqueness, instrumentalization, harmfulness, lives lived in the shadow of another, and the alleged right to genetic ignorance. She finds that none of these objections could justify a total ban on cloning, if the procedure could be made safe for the children born and the women involved. The catch, as she sees it, is that cloning cannot be made safe without research into it, and research into it cannot in the foreseeable future be accepted due to the practice's being unsafe. Her conclusion is, consequently, that while there would be nothing intrinsically wrong in the successful reproductive cloning of humans, we do not currently have ethically acceptable means to guarantee its success.

In chapter six, Louise Irving challenges some of the main philosophical and legal arguments that have been employed to defend the legalization of international organ sales. Her view is that, on the surface, all the current bans on the practice are founded almost exclusively on people's feelings of disgust and indignation, which is why liberal philosophical and legal thinking forces us to the permissive conclusion. She argues, however, that since these ways of thinking rely on an inadequate, "negative" concept of freedom and autonomy, we should question the demand for rationality, and the foundation of prevailing laws, rather than the views people so widely hold. A more "positive" notion of liberty would, according to her, recognize the values supported by respect for liberty, and also identify some elements of humanity which cannot be legitimately alienated.

4. Facts, Ideals, and Approaches

In the next three chapters, the focus is on empirical facts, moral ideals, and their relationship, as well as on the ways in which we can seek knowledge concerning them in bioethics and neighboring fields. More specifically, the topics include the gap between facts and values in bioethics, the ideal and reality of informed consent in medicine, and the lessons to be learned from empirical business ethics.

In chapter seven, Eve Garrard and Stephen Wilkinson turn their attention to the role of the natural and social sciences in bioethical research. They acknowledge the relevance of facts produced by both to ethical inquiries, but contend that these facts, or their production, is not part of bioethics properly conceived. Biology and medicine can reveal causal connections between our actions and the outcomes of those actions to ourselves and others, but they cannot solve ethical problems, because the causal connections in question do not contain within themselves labels as to their goodness or badness, rightness or wrongness. Similarly, they argue, sociological studies can provide information about the social reception and consequences of our political decisions, but they cannot enlighten us as to the reasonableness, and hence morality, of people's responses.

In chapter eight, Angus Dawson questions the prevailing insistence on informed consent in the face of empirical reality. He concentrates on the idea that to be informed or valid, people's consent to medical procedures and research programmes should ideally be based on adequate information concerning these procedures and programmes. This is one of the basic requirements of the principle, and unless it is met, the benefits that are supposed to flow from its observance in terms of autonomy and well-being remain unclear. Sociological studies seem to suggest, however, that most people do not understand or remember the things professionals tell them before they are asked to sign the relevant forms. Dawson notes that the difficulties involved are so pervasive that a mere call for better communication skills on the part of practitioners is not enough any more.

In chapter nine, Søren Holm compares empirical studies conducted in business and healthcare ethics. In the former, the empirical strand is better established, and some research into the moral dimensions of executive decision making seems to aim at, and succeed in, actually building a body of knowledge on which further studies can be based. This is not yet the case in bioethics, where almost every new project starts from new methodological premises. Another deficiency in empirical healthcare ethics is that the immorality of professionals and their activities is seldom examined. The phenomenon of corruption has been the focus of several studies in business ethics, whereas bribing and similar practices in medicine have been barely touched. Yet it would be useful to know whether backhanders and sloppy practices in fact facilitate the provision of healthcare or hinder it.

5. Responsibility and Risk Taking

The next two chapters are dedicated to responsibility and risk taking in corporate decision making and other economic activities. These contributions continue the discussion on the interface between bioethics and business ethics, and show how a proper grasp of the concepts employed in economic debates is in many cases essential for the understanding of bioethical issues as well.

In chapter ten, Jukka Kilpi sketches a model of corporate responsibility. He stresses the importance of background ethical theories, and defines corporations as networks of contracts between rationally self-interested parties. Corporations, thus defined, can be assigned responsibilities which are based on the utility and morality of keeping the promises that underlie legally binding contracts. The moral responsibility of corporations and their representatives can, Kilpi argues, be extended to cover the interests of stakeholders as well as shareholders, as all these participate in one way or another in the contractual network. While businesses can and should, according to Kilpi, be motivated by their self-interest and profits, the assumption of strict product liability would add an element of caution to the proceedings and ensure the protection of everybody's vital interests.

In chapter eleven, Peter Lucas challenges the use of cost-benefit analyses and other economic appraisal methods in healthcare decision making. His challenge is based on the observation that all economic assessments of this kind rely on a particular attitude toward the desirable and undesirable consequences of our choices: namely, risk neutrality. A risk neutral agent chooses the option which is most likely to maximize net benefits, regardless of the size and nature of the promises and dangers involved. Economic appraisal methods standardly assume that risk neutrality is the only rational approach to risk. Lucas argues, however, that the alternative strategies of risk aversion and risk preferring can be equally rational under conditions of considerable uncertainty, for instance, conditions under which healthcare decisions are usually made.

6. Educational Concerns

In the three concluding chapters of the book, the authors concentrate on the moral progress and character development of nurses and physicians, and on the theories underlying bioethical reflection. In keeping with the European ethical tradition, virtues, duties, and consequences are all addressed as fundamental elements of professional morality.

In chapter twelve, Simon Woods studies the nature of moral progress in healthcare students and professionals. Considering the case of Mrs Gamp, a far-from-ideal nurse from Charles Dickens's *Martin Chuzzlewit*, he argues that there are certain developments which can reasonably be seen as signs of moral progress in novice nurses. These include an understanding of the situation from a moral point of view, an awareness of the special relationship between a carer and the cared-for, and an ability to assess one's own responses and working methods in a professional situation. Any changes we can perceive in professionals to these directions can, Woods argues, be regarded as instances of moral progress, in spite of the acute difficulties we face if we set out to define more generally the essence and mechanics of ethical improvement in the human race.

In chapter thirteen, Mark Sheehan delineates "a kind of" virtue ethics for physicians. He starts by considering the notion of a practice which develops socially and which has its own distinctive ends, or internal goods. He argues that it is possible to build a teleological model of professional morality on the practice of medicine by "physicians in the strict sense."

These theoretical entities cannot be mistaken, they do not earn money, and they always seek only to benefit their patients. Both actual and ideal instances of medicine can add to or subtract from this formula, but the metaethics of medical practice can, Sheehan maintains, best be based on this idea. What physicians in the strict sense do when they form professional relationships with their patients and apply their skills to the care of those patients defines what the virtues of medical practice are.

In chapter fourteen, Peter Herissone-Kelly considers the situation of a bioethicist who hovers between a belief in the importance of consequences and a conviction that the rights of individuals should be respected for their own sake. He constructs a non-utilitarian version of consequentialism, which states that in choosing our actions and inactions we should always aim to maximize the number of people whose rights come to be respected as a result. While this solution satisfies the consequence-awareness of his imaginary bioethicist, it seems to fall short of respecting individuals as their own persons. However, Herissone-Kelly argues that this has little practical impact, as people who make policy decisions have no way of respecting the rights of individuals against those of other individuals anyway. Rights claims seem to fail when they are most needed.

7. Blessed Confusion?

Philosophically speaking, the conflicting views expressed and competing claims made in the chapters of this book convey an important message. Reality, be it physical, moral, or social, is not something to be taken for granted. Its ontological status can be whatever it is, but our knowledge and understanding of it will probably always be more or less messy.

When we realize this, we can react in at least two ways. We can maintain that good and bad, right and wrong are socially-constructed categories, which can only be re-negotiated through political struggle. Or we can insist that academic studies can shed at least some light on ethical matters. Either way, there still seem to be things to be done by bioethicists.

NOTES

1. Georg Wilhelm Friedrich Hegel, *Hegel's Philosophy of Right*, trans. by T. M. Knox (Oxford: Oxford University Press, 1967), § 182 ff.

One

THE CASE OF BACK-STREET ABORTION

Harry Lesser

1. The Argument from Back-Street Abortion

An important example of the use of empirical facts in healthcare ethics occurs in what may be called "the argument from back-street abortion," which has been used both in arguments for legalizing abortion, and in arguments for maintaining its legality, whether on demand or subject to various limitations. It is the argument that the result of criminalizing abortion is that, whether or not the total number of abortions is decreased (which may be held to be uncertain), the decrease is certainly slight, while the number of unskilled and unhygienic abortions is certainly increased. So, the argument continues, even if we firmly believe abortion to be wrong, we must admit that to make it altogether illegal, or very difficult to obtain legally, does appreciably more harm than good. It is by no means the only argument for legal abortion, but it is the only one that is addressed to those who firmly believe that abortion is morally wrong, by presenting an empirical fact, or set of facts, and arguing that given these facts—given the empirical consequences of making abortion illegal—we should be prepared to legalize it, irrespective of whether it is morally right or wrong.

As a result, the "argument from back-street abortion" has been widely used, and can be found quite frequently in both formal and informal discussions of the rights and wrongs of abortion, whether verbal or written: possibly it was the really decisive argument in getting a change in the law in the United Kingdom. This chapter will be concerned with its use as a conclusive argument, with the view that this empirical fact—I will assume that it is a fact, and that, although this cannot be quantified, one effect of preventing legal abortion is to increase back-street abortion and therefore to increase unskilled and unhygienic abortion—is all that is required to settle the question whether abortion should be legally available. As an example of the argument, I will take a short passage from an account of nursing during the Second World War, Monica Dickens's *One Pair of Feet*,[1] in which she gives her reaction to having as a patient a woman, "Irene," who had been nearly killed by a botched abortion, and who was left unable to have any more children. I will return to this passage, but for the moment just quote it:

> Before I was a nurse I was not in favour of legal abortion. Now I think that anything would be preferable to some of the ghastly things that are perpetrated outside the law. If women could see what some of their sex

have to go through in consequence, nightmare old women in basement flats would lose their trade.

2. The First Element in the Argument: The Law Should Reflect Actual Positive Morality

The first thing to notice is that there can be up to four different elements in this argument, not all present in the above quotation, but not incompatible with each other. The existence, or potential existence, of back-street abortion could be seen as showing that:

- to make abortion illegal is contrary to our actual morality, as opposed to our official moralizing;
- it results in unregulated abortion, which is in itself a bad thing;
- it is largely ineffective, because abortion, like private sexual behavior, is the kind of thing the law cannot significantly prevent but can only drive underground;
- the harm done by unskilled operators outweighs the benefit of reducing the total number of abortions, even if this happens.

It is also worth noting that the argument, with the exception of the last point, has sometimes been extended to euthanasia, with the suggestion being made that we have in effect a situation of "back-street euthanasia," in which euthanasia is regularly carried out, admittedly mostly by medically qualified people, but illegally and entirely unregulated. This will not be my concern here, but I want to examine the four elements in the argument in turn.

The first element comes from the view that the law ought to reflect existing morality, whatever it is, and that it is a mistake to prohibit what is widely believed not to be wrong, or to punish any crime with what is seen as excessive severity. (In early nineteenth century England the widespread use of the death penalty had the consequence that juries often refused to convict.) This was argued, for example, by C. S. Lewis. In a paper reprinted in *Personal Concerns*,[2] Lewis says that if we ceased to disapprove of murder we should no doubt be both fools and villains, but it would be better to admit the fact than to have a law against murder that was habitually disregarded, and juries who acquitted murderers whatever the evidence. The question is whether this should apply as a general principle, or only when the effect of the separation of law and morality is to make the law largely ineffective.

Thus it might be held that there is no sense in imposing severe penalties to deter crime if a consequence of their severity is that juries refuse to convict and criminals are not punished at all: it is a historical fact that a petition to have stealing from a bleaching ground removed from the list of capital offences was made by the owners of bleaching grounds, who were understandably bothered by the invariable acquittals of those charged with this offense. On the other hand, not every law that lacks general moral backing has this consequence. It is very likely that the laws against race discrimination and incitement to racial hatred would, if put to a referendum, have failed to command majority support, but they have played some part in altering the general moral view of what is acceptable, even though more needs to be done. Similarly, the outlawing of corporal punishment, even in very mild forms, in countries such as Sweden, was a conscious and largely successful move to alter general attitudes. We might, I think, therefore conclude that, with regard to abortion, the pure fact, if it is a fact, that most people in our society, including many Roman Catholics, do not regard it as always wrong, is not, considered in isolation, a sufficient ground for legalizing it, inasmuch as exactly the same argument could be applied to racial discrimination, in earlier days at any rate. What is to the point, however, is whether one consequence of this is that any law against abortion is bound to be ineffective. This will be considered later.

One point, though, that should be considered briefly, is what constitutes the actual morality, the "positive morality" of a society. I am assuming that this should be defined by what people in practice tolerate and encourage, whether or not this is in line with official pronouncements, or with what they feel constrained to say on official occasions: what people do is evidence, but cannot define their morality, because it is so normal to act against our own moral standards. For example, until well into the last century, official sexual morality held that pre-marital sex was wrong, while actual morality held that it was wrong for women but permissible up to a point for men—there are problems with this position, which creates an ideal of conduct that is among other things physically impossible, but it was the actual morality of the time. And it is quite arguable that even at that time abortion was largely seen as something not to be lightly undertaken but sometimes permissible or even necessary. Certainty is lacking and, as often in this area, much of the evidence is anecdotal, though evidence from many sources is available. Nevertheless, if the argument so far is correct, the crucial issue is that of effectiveness.

3. Back-Street Abortion as Unregulated

Before considering effectiveness, we need to consider the second element in the argument. This is the point that back-street abortion, unlike legalized abortion, is necessarily unregulated, so that issues of who is to be allowed an abortion and how it is to be performed are decided in ways that are entirely unprincipled, depending on who a woman happens to know, how much money she can raise, and so on, with no reference to morality, social policy, or medical advisability. It is true that legalizing abortion did not eliminate arbitrariness, probably caused partly by the virtual impossibility of framing the law with precision and partly by the differing moral attitudes among senior medical staff, which had the consequence that for many years after the change in the law that allowed abortion for a range of social and medical reasons, it was well known that it was much easier to obtain an abortion in some areas of the United Kingdom than others. But even this was at least the result of genuine disagreement on a matter of principle, instead of, as previously, the result of there being in practice one law for the rich and one for the poor.

So this part of the argument amounts to saying that if abortion is illegal it will still take place, but considerations of morality and justice will not affect whether and how it is carried out: indeed principles of any kind will be excluded. The argument consequently depends on showing that the law is ineffective. Even if this can be shown, someone who regarded abortion as wrong in principle might take the view that we cannot sensibly raise questions about the "just distribution" of what ought not to be distributed in the first place. If abortions ought not to be performed, restricting them arbitrarily to the well-off is no worse than restricting them on what they regard as misplaced social grounds. It may even be seen as at least having the merit of reducing the overall number of abortions.

4. The Effectiveness of Laws against Abortion

The crucial point thus appears to be effectiveness. There are some obvious problems in deciding this issue. First, the notion itself is vague. All laws are sometimes disobeyed. How much disobedience is needed for us to regard the law as in reality non-operative, or close to non-operative? Second, there is the problem of information. Although back-street abortionists need publicity of a kind in order to carry on their business, they do not publish annual statistics of the numbers of operations they have carried out! But there are serious grounds for arguing that in this area the law, though it may reduce the total number of abortions carried out, has really quite little effect. The argument would be that, even when abortion is illegal and there are a few prosecutions now and again, it is always possible for any woman to obtain an abortion, with little risk of prosecution, provided that she is sufficiently determined and able to raise the money for the fee. And this appears to be generally true, instead of true in some societies and not others, because of the nature of the operation, which can fairly easily be kept secret, and because it is very hard, without an eyewitness, to prove that a woman has had an abortion rather than a miscarriage. What cannot be guaranteed, when abortion is illegal, is a safe and hygienic abortion, unless the woman in question has access to sufficient financial resources.

I would therefore suggest that there is evidence that in the ordinary sense of the word, the law against abortion was not effective in the United Kingdom, and probably not elsewhere. Does it automatically follow from this empirical fact that abortion ought not to be a crime, or at any rate that it should be legal under some circumstances? Two replies might be made to this suggestion. The first is that what has just been argued does not show that the law was totally ineffective. Its effect may still have been to produce some decrease in the numbers of abortions. It appears likely, after all, given the high number of legal abortions after the law changed, that legalization was responsible for some increase, although we cannot be quite certain about this, given that the number of previous illegal abortions is unknown. If there was an increase after legalization, it is reasonable to think that the previous law had some deterrent effect, although no doubt other factors, such as the general change in moral attitudes at that time, also played a part in bringing about the increase. So we might conclude, though not with certainty, that the law had some effect, albeit a pretty small one. And a convinced opponent of abortion might argue that this was enough to justify it: if abortion is murder, the prevention of a single abortion would be enough to justify the law.

Second, the convinced anti-abortionist might argue that there is a need for a society to declare itself to be against abortion by maintaining a law against it, regardless of effectiveness. This would be the reverse of the argument considered earlier, that the law should reflect existing morality; instead, the argument would be that the law should give a moral lead. The objection to this would be that this could be justified only if the law were at least in line with a social trend, so that there was a reasonable chance of its becoming in time both effective and acceptable, as has partly happened in the two examples above, of race discrimination here and of corporal punishment in Sweden and some other countries. But where the law is out of line with existing morality and the signs are that the gap is going to widen, as was the case here, then maintaining a hypocritical and ineffective law serves no good purpose. So this reply from the anti-abortionist can be rejected, but the first reply still holds.

5. The Bad Consequences of Making Abortion Criminal

The argument that any law prohibiting abortion will be largely ineffective is thus a strong one, but anyone convinced that abortion is murder, or simply that it is morally wrong, could still reply that even a small decrease in the number of abortions is worthwhile. To answer this we will have to bring in the final element in the "argument from back-street abortion," the argument that even if there is this beneficial consequence of the law, it must be outweighed by the harm done by unskilled abortionists working in unhygienic conditions outside the law. This argument can be presented in two slightly different ways, which are not mutually exclusive.

In its first form the argument points to a whole range of bad consequences that follow from making abortion illegal. The most important is the encouragement given to unskilled and unscrupulous abortionists working outside the normal medical framework, resulting at worst in death or permanent injury, but also in many other evils—financial exploitation, the general injustice of "one law for the rich, one for the poor," difficulties in providing any psychological support or advice for the women in question, the problems caused by people being recommended unreliable and dangerous "home remedies." We should also note that one consequence of abortion being illegal was that there could not be open seeking of advice as to whether to have a pregnancy terminated, with the result that some women who might under those circumstances have decided against termination ended up having abortions, so that the effect of illegality is not always toward reduction of abortion. But essentially the argument would be that a possible slight reduction in numbers, even if seen as a gain, is easily outweighed by the sometimes permanent injuries, danger, physical and mental suffering, injustice, and even deaths caused by criminalization.

The other form of the argument is the one used in effect by Monica Dickens in the passage quoted earlier, that criminalization has particular consequences that are so horrible that allowing abortion, even in increased numbers, has to be better than allowing them to happen. This argument might be dismissed as emotive, but, I think, wrongly. If we are arguing for a particular policy we must take account properly of its consequences, as shown for example in the case of "Irene," as Monica Dickens calls the patient whose situation caused her to make these comments. Not every distressing detail of Irene's case is relevant. It is irrelevant to this particular argument that Irene had originally wanted the baby and let her boyfriend talk her into an abortion, or that the aborted fetus was brought to the hospital with her, or that she was put in a labor ward, surrounded by other people's babies and now unable ever to have one of her own. All these are reasons for feeling sorry for Irene, but not reasons for changing the law. But it is highly relevant that it was the law that prevented her from having a relatively safe abortion, with the result that she had a horribly bungled one. And it is therefore a fair argument that the inevitable harm done to her and others, even if they are a minority among those given illegal abortions, is a sufficient reason for not making abortion illegal, as Monica Dickens argues. It is also a live argument: what happened to Irene is less likely to happen now than in the early 1940s, even in an illegal operation, but it still could, and if illegal operations became widespread no doubt sometimes it would. Termination of a pregnancy is much safer now than it was in the 1940s, but the means to make it safe would not necessarily be available to illegal operators, even if they were concerned with safety, which itself cannot be guaranteed.

6. The Anti-Abortionist's Reply

Despite all this, the anti-abortionist could make no fewer than four replies to this argument, in either of its forms. These are (with apologies for being so schematic):

- The makers and enforcers of the law are in no way morally responsible for the voluntary actions of those who break it: no one forces anyone either to carry out or to undergo an illegal abortion, whether hygienic or unhygienic.
- The calculation has not been done properly, because one also has to reckon in the way in which legalization has produced a "culture of abortion" and started a "slippery slope" that has led from allowing abortion for good reasons, medical or social, to allowing abortion on demand, and will end with infanticide.
- Abortion is in itself so wicked that the reduction in numbers, however small, produced by criminalization, is enough to outweigh all the bad consequences.
- It is wrong to make calculations at all with regard to an action such as abortion or murder: it must simply be forbidden.

The first of these replies does not, I think, hold up. It is presumably true that the legislator is not morally responsible for what people do in disobedience to the law. But it is also true that legislators, in considering whether any particular activity should be legal or illegal, are obliged to take into account, as best they can, which situation is the less bad, and to avoid making any activity a crime if the consequences are worse than if it were legal. They cannot ignore that it is illegality that makes back-street abortion profitable, and simply say that no one is forced into it. The second point is, I think, empirically refutable. It is true that the incidence of abortion has probably risen since it was legalized, and that some of this rise is due to its being more easily available. But it is not clear that the rise is that large, given the previous amount of illegal abortion, or that other factors, such as the general change in attitudes, are not equally important. There are also two reasons to deny that there has been a slippery slope to abortion on demand. One is that the restrictions in the law are in practice unworkable, and the other is that there were from the start many doctors who were determined to act in accordance with the decision of the individual patient rather than the exact legal technicalities—we have not gone from using the law, with all its limitations on when abortion is permissible, to ignoring it, but instead its distinctions have been found unworkable from the beginning. Moreover, not every development has been a relaxation. As the age of viability has moved earlier, so also have the restrictions on late abortions tightened. Finally, there has been no attempt of any kind to legalize infanticide.

This leaves the last two replies. Though the reasoning is different in each case, both amount to saying that reducing the amount of abortion "trumps" avoiding the harm caused by criminalizing it. On one view, this is because the harm prevented, even if it amounts to a small lowering of the abortion rate, outweighs the harm done by the measures needed to prevent it. On the other view, it is because there is a moral imperative to prevent abortion, which is not open to being overridden by utilitarian considerations. How do we assess these, and what does this show about the question with which we started: are the empirical facts about back-street abortion enough to establish that abortion, irrespective of whether it is morally wrong, ought to be legal? (I leave aside the possibility of legalizing it on some grounds but not others, which, if what was said above is correct, is probably in practice unworkable, but assume there will be some limit on the number of weeks into the pregnancy at which it is allowable or normally allowable.) And does all this show anything about the status of empirical claims in general, in the area of healthcare ethics?

It does show one thing that, I think, is important. If a law is ineffective, or would be ineffective, and this can be shown empirically, that law should not be passed, or should be repealed. This is one case in which the empirical evidence is sufficient to determine action, but the evidence itself is often not easy to obtain. But there is a problem with a case like this one, where there is, probably, a quite limited effectiveness. Many people would see the effectiveness as being too low to justify the law, or would see it as outweighed by the amount of harm produced by the law. But if they do not, what answer can be made? Can we appeal to reasonableness, or is this also contestable? Will what is reasonable to one person be seen by another as an abandonment of principle?

We should also note that there is some artificiality in treating this issue in isolation. The person still in favor of making abortion a crime may also wish to change social institutions and values so that life is made easier for single parents—and "Irene" would not need to go to an abortionist in the first place. The person in favor of legal abortion may also wish to improve contraception and its availability, and the availability of advice, so that again fewer people seek abortions. But in the end there appears to be an unavoidable dispute about values. Both sides agree that abortion, considered in itself, is an evil: we have been considering the specific argument that abortion should be legal whether it is wrong or not, rather than the questions of whether it is wrong or who should decide. But some people hold that unhygienic and unskilled abortion is so much worse than abortion itself that it is preferable to allow more abortion of a safer kind; others may hold that it is always right to reduce the incidence of abortion, even at this cost.

My conclusion at the moment would be this. With regard to issues of what laws it is right to have, and what conduct should be outlawed, an empirical demonstration that a law is, or would be, ineffective, should be a conclusive reason against having that law. But if the demonstration shows only that the effectiveness is quite limited or at a cost, even a heavy cost, the matter is then still contestable. It turns crucially on how wrong we believe abortion to be, not simply on whether we believe it to be wrong. Whatever our beliefs, we must consider quite carefully the empirical evidence, and this includes not just facts and figures, but facing what happens to people like Irene. For many people this settles the matter, but for it to do so we must make a decision about values as well as an empirical decision. Nevertheless, what also, I hope, emerges from this discussion is the extreme importance of the empirical, of finding out, as best we can, what actually happens and what the likely effects of the different options are. And crucially, this does also show that, even if the empirical evidence does not settle the matter, there is a clear obligation to discover what it is. The anti-abortionist can claim that the considerations raised by cases such as Irene's should be overridden, but cannot legitimately claim that they are irrelevant.

NOTES

1. Monica Dickens, *One Pair of Feet* (London: Penguin, 1956), p. 196.
2. C. S. Lewis, *Personal Concerns* (Glasgow: Collins, 1986), pp. 105–6.

Two

SUICIDE, SELF-SACRIFICE, AND THE DUTY TO DIE

Doris Schroeder

1. "Duty to Die?"

Most philosophical literature on "suicide" examines the following questions. Is suicide morally indefensible (Thomas Aquinas, Saint Augustine, Immanuel Kant, Ludwig Wittgenstein) or morally permissible (Seneca, David Hume)? How can suicide be defined (Emile Durkheim)? And how can suicide be marked off from other types of self-caused deaths? I am interested in this last question, particularly the distinction between suicide on the one hand, and self-sacrifice, with its connotations of altruism, on the other. For instance, Maximilian Kolbe, a Franciscan monk and priest, substituted himself for a father at Auschwitz. He took the place of his fellow prisoner who was condemned to death by starvation, but eventually died from a fatal injection on 14 August 1941. By this heroic act, Kolbe brought about his own death intentionally, but he is not usually classified as a suicide.[1]

The distinction between suicide and self-sacrifice is important as it leads to my main question, namely: how does self-sacrifice relate to physician-assisted suicide? Could we ever reasonably talk of physician-assisted self-sacrifice? Literature dealing with physician-assisted suicide defines the "relevant pool [of people who might benefit as] . . . the class of persons who will be patients suffering from a terminal or incurable, intractable illness, who will be competent."[2] It is this class of people from whom occasionally a duty to die is demanded. According to Euripides, patients with long illnesses ought "when they no longer serve the land . . . quit this life."[3] Friedrich Nietzsche believed that "the sick are parasites on society [for whom] . . . under certain conditions it is indecent to continue living."[4] More recently a United States governor was widely quoted to have said that the elderly, irreversibly ill, who need substantial medical resources, have a "duty to die."[5] And, perhaps most importantly, John Hardwig, Professor in the Clinical Ethics Program at East Tennessee State University, explicitly promoted a duty to die in the *Hastings Center Report*.[6] How this demand could be analyzed philosophically with the notion of self-sacrifice will be the focus of this chapter.

To this end, three topics will be discussed. First, where can the line be drawn between suicide and self-sacrifice? Second, what are the main differences between suicide and physician-assisted suicide? Third, is physician-assisted self-sacrifice possible or morally desirable?

2. Suicide and Altruism

Emile Durkheim defined suicide as "death resulting directly or indirectly from a positive or negative act of the victim himself which he knows will produce this result."[7] The definition has since been criticized as being too broad.[8] However, before we look at its limitations, we should explicate which cases of suicide Durkheim rightly captures with his definition. The elements needed to make sense of Durkheim's definition are: death, causal chain (direct or indirect), victim's action (including negative acts or, in other words, omissions) and foreknowledge. The following case will illustrate these elements.

James skis in the Alps in April in an area cordoned off by the *Bergwacht* due to imminently expected avalanches. He passes the barricades and ignores the warning signs. The act under consideration is skiing in this area. *Direct causal chain between act and death*: A snow plank avalanche hits James and he dies within minutes from injuries and breathing problems. *Indirect causal chain between act and death*: An ice avalanche hits James and throws him into a glacier, where he dies, physically unharmed, from hypothermia. *Positive act*: James enters the avalanche area, despite the sounds of approaching avalanches. He dies. *Negative act*: James does not leave the avalanche area, despite the sounds of approaching avalanches. He dies. *Foreknowledge*: In all of the above permutations, James is aware that avalanches can kill and he is aware that the area he skis in will—in all likelihood—see avalanches within the next hour.

According to Durkheim's definition, James is a suicide but the following would not count as suicide. *No causal chain between act and death*: Before meeting an avalanche, James is hit by a huge ibex, his skis fail to come off, and he dies from injuries inflicted by the fall. *No foreknowledge*: James is a novice skier, unaware of the dangers of avalanches and unable to read the warning signs. Foreknowledge and causal chain certainly seem to be necessary conditions for suicide (in addition to action and death), but are they sufficient conditions?

At least one feature seems to be missing from the above definition, namely the agent's intention. Durkheim purposefully left out all mental concepts such as intention and motives for action when defining suicide. He wanted to arrive at a "scientific" definition of suicide, and clearly to demarcate his research from research in psychology.[9] However, it has been argued that two types of self-caused deaths both related to intention must be eliminated from Durkheim's group, namely those based on purely altruistic actions as well as those forced by outsiders. According to William Tolhurst, Durkheim's definition is too broad as it wrongly calls self-caused deaths with overwhelming altruistic or morally praiseworthy features suicides.[10] James could have been a member of the *Bergwacht* searching for survivors of previous avalanches. So far as Tolhurst is concerned, this would not make him a suicide. Likewise, Tom Beauchamp argues that Durkheim's definition is too broad, because it does not distinguish between uncoerced and coerced self-deaths—the latter should not be classified as suicides.[11] James could have been forced onto the ski slope by an armed maniac who gave him a choice: either I will shoot you, or you show that you can escape an avalanche. Given that death is more certain in the former case, James decides to take the chance.

In this chapter, I will concentrate on altruism and suicide. Is there a fundamental difference between self-sacrifice and suicide, the defining element of which is altruism? Why should James not be classed as a suicide even if he is in the avalanche area as a *Bergwacht* member? There are three reasons why we might want to differentiate between suicide and self-sacrifice. First, for a considerable number of thinkers, mostly from religious backgrounds, suicide has negative moral connotations, whilst self-sacrifice has not.[12] So, we might not want to call Maximilian Kolbe (canonized in 1982) a "suicide." Second, it is the aim of some Western philosophy to define concepts as precisely as possible in order to facilitate communication and understanding. If there is a conceptual difference between suicide and self-sacrifice, it is worth bringing out for the sake of analysis and to stimulate further debate. Third, ethicists might want to analyze the concept of self-sacrifice, regardless of death, and this analysis should be compatible with the concept as developed in suicide debates. Kolbe died in 1941. However, an alternative scenario is conceivable in which his life was saved by Allied troops liberating Auschwitz. Would his act have been any less morally praiseworthy, had he been awakened from near-death by an Allied doctor?

For the purpose of this chapter, altruism will, following the *Oxford English Dictionary*, be defined as the "practice of disinterested and selfless concern for the well-being of others." A straightforward and simple strategy suggests itself if we want to distinguish self-sacrifice from suicide: namely, to use the doctrine of double effect. In order to clarify this, let us look at some examples:

- As far as we know, Maximilian Kolbe wanted to save his Jewish fellow prisoner from death, and accepted his own death as an unavoidable consequence. It is reasonable to assume that he did not want to die, or that he might even have hoped not to die ("perhaps my church will intervene on my behalf"; "perhaps the Nazis will not let an Aryan starve to death," and so on).
- If James was forced by an armed maniac onto the slope, he was trying to avoid certain death by gun, whilst accepting potential death from avalanche as a possible consequence.

- If James was on the slope as a *Bergwacht* member, he wanted to rescue potential survivors from a previous avalanche, whilst acknowledging that he might be killed in the process.
- The pilot of a disabled plane does not use her parachute and remains in her plane to prevent it from crashing in a populated area.[13] Her main intention is to avoid death, but not her own, which she accepts as a probably unavoidable consequence.
- A soldier covers a grenade with his body in order to protect his comrades. He thereby accepts almost certain death in order to save others.

One feature these examples have in common is that the main intention is characterized by "disinterested and selfless concern for the well-being of others" (see above) and can therefore be called "altruistic." Hence, very pragmatically and straightforwardly, suicide and self-sacrifice could be distinguished as follows: a suicide intends her own death, whilst a self-sacrificer intends the outcome of an action, which can be characterized as altruistic, but only accepts death as an unavoidable but unwanted consequence. Hence, death is the main aim of a suicide, but only a foreseen possibility in the case of the self-sacrificer.

There are borderline cases, where people using the distinction might not be able to agree, and these are of specific interest for this chapter. For instance, Captain Oates can be considered both a suicide and a self-sacrificer. Oates was a polar explorer and a member of the Scott team. Upon falling ill during an expedition, he walked out into a blizzard at night in order to avoid becoming a burden to his friends (self-sacrifice). On the other hand, he must have aimed for death itself (suicide), as he would have put his friends into an even worse position had they assumed he could have been alive and aimed to get him back.

One could argue that he would not have objected had aliens rescued him and returned him to a hospital in his country, as his main purpose (not being a burden to his friends) would still be satisfied. However, if we have to go to such lengths for an argument, we might as well argue that, had aliens taken away their feelings of tiredness of life (*Lebensmüdigkeit*), Stefan Zweig, Ernest Hemingway, Paul Celan, and so on, would still have wanted to live and can therefore not be called suicides.

So, at this stage we could say that Oates's death represents a mixed case, an overlap between the sets of suicides and self-sacrificers, which shows that they cannot be distinguished without gray areas. Some people would call him a suicide, others a self-sacrificer.

However, applying the above definition has one major disadvantage, namely that it asks: does the person in question want to commit suicide? Does she aim for death for death's sake or for other reasons? So, we are begging the question. In my opinion, there are three possible ways to deal with this problem. First, we stay with a "scientific" version of defining suicide, following Durkheim, and end up with an enormous domain of suicides and a zero-domain of self-sacrificers. Second, we can claim that it is impossible to reach a rigorous definition of suicide and self-sacrifice. Third, we end up with a reasonable definition but beg the question and use mental concepts in the process.

Against using mental concepts, it could be argued that primary motives can never be established. Perhaps Socrates was a suicide who cleverly engineered his death. Perhaps Kolbe was tired of life in the concentration camp (although death by starvation is probably not the most likely course for those who want to commit suicide). It is possible, but the empirical impossibility of establishing primary motives should not discourage us from finding conceptual boundaries. Although we may never be sure about actual events, there is a distinctive difference between a soldier who throws himself onto a live grenade to save his comrades, and a soldier who trips and falls onto the grenade with the same results. So, for the remainder of this chapter, option three will be chosen and its limitations accepted.

3. Suicide and Physician-Assisted Suicide

Could the distinction between suicides and self-sacrificers be applied to debates about physician-assisted suicide? Would a "duty to die" for the intractably sick—as advocated by Colorado's former Governor Richard Lamm, Hardwig, Nietzsche, and Euripides—amount to a duty to self-sacrifice assisted by physicians? To answer this question, it is necessary to define both concepts. Based on the above, suicide will be understood as death resulting directly or indirectly from a *strongly intended* positive or negative act of the victim herself, which she knows will produce this result (italics added to Durkheim's definition). Self-sacrifice requires the main intention to show extraordinarily selfless concern for the well-being of others, and only foresight of one's own unwanted death as a consequence.

Physician-assisted suicide will be taken to mean a facilitation of suicide by physicians who "provide the knowledge and/or the means by which a patient can take her own life."[14] The amount of help provided can range from giving information only, to major involvement in setting up suitable equipment. For instance, the German Society for Humane Dying (*Deutsche Gesellschaft für humanes Sterben*) used to provide a booklet entitled "Dignified and Responsible Death" (*Menschenwürdiges und selbstverantwortliches Sterben*) to members under certain conditions. The leaflet gave information about prescription drugs, how to obtain them, what dosage would be lethal, and how to avoid complications such as vomiting (suicide and assisted suicide are legal in Germany; euthanasia is not). When Australia's Northern Territory province briefly legalized euthanasia and physician-assisted suicide in 1996, one possibility for patients was to end their life by obtaining a lethal injection after initiating the process via computer controls. The injection was not given by a doctor but automatically administered through a previously installed injection channel. So, this was a case of physician-assisted suicide rather than euthanasia, according to the standard distinction. In euthanasia cases, "the physician performs the last causal step leading to the death of the patient, and thus can be said to kill the patient."[15] In cases of physician-assisted suicide, the patient performs this last causal step.[16]

What are the main relevant differences between suicide and physician-assisted suicide here? (I shall concentrate on standard rather than unusual cases of each, and exclude suicides that are set up to fail: so-called "cry-for-help" suicides.)

Suicide	**Physician-Assisted Suicide**
Very private, individualistic act, which requires only one person.	Less private, less individualistic act, which requires at least two parties.
Full self-sufficiency of suicidal person given.	Partial self-sufficiency requires in-volvement of physician.
Standardised, sociologically est-ablished reasons for suicide are manifold.[17]	Reasons for physician-assisted sui-cide are mostly pain, suffering and perceived or prospective loss of dignity amongst the incurably ill.[18]

4. Physician-Assisted Suicide and Altruism

Physician-assisted self-sacrifices would have to satisfy the following three conditions:

- Death facilitated by physicians (providing the knowledge or the means by which a patient can take her own life).
- Death foreseen as the direct or indirect result of a positive or negative act of the victim herself, which she knows will produce this result.
- The main intention behind the act shows extraordinarily selfless concern for the well-being of others.

A particular case study might clarify the requirements (from the *Hastings Center Report*,[19] based on fact but edited to preserve confidentiality). Gary Davidson, a twenty-eight year old gay man, was hospitalized with pneumonia, having been diagnosed as suffering from AIDS one week earlier. Mr Davidson refused treatment for pneumonia supported by his family and his lover, arguing that "he did not deserve to take up a bed in the hospital and continue to receive medical treatment that could better benefit another patient."[20]

The case is not unrepresentative. According to Joanne Lynn (Director of the Center to Improve Care of the Dying) and Felicia Cohn (Director of the Program in Bioethics at the George Washington University Medical Center), "patients often say, 'I just don't want to be a burden,' and they mean it, emotionally, physically, and financially."[21]

At first sight, Mr Davidson might be regarded as fulfilling the above criteria, and as agreeing with Euripides', Nietzsche's, Hardwig's, and Lamm's demands. His death would be facilitated by doctors, who would have to stop treating him. According to R. G. Frey,[22] it depends on the legal situation whether withdrawal of treatment counts as suicide or physician-assisted suicide. With a firm legal right to refuse treatment in place, we would speak of suicide. However, if we rely on the physician's co-operation to withdraw treatment without a firm right, we ought to speak of physician-assisted suicide. So, death would result directly from a negative act of the patient, Mr Davidson, and his doctors who know that the act will produce this result. The intention as communicated to the doctors shows extraordinarily selfless concern for the well-being of others (not wanting to take away medical resources).

This could be regarded as the prototypical case of physician-assisted self-sacrifice (if it exists), as those who are in the group who possibly "qualify" for physician-assisted suicide are overwhelmingly patients with a serious illness. In addition, their main altruistic contribution, from a purely economic point of view, would be to save medical resources for others.

However, there seems to be a distinctive difference between the case of Gary Davidson and the case of Maximilian Kolbe. Kolbe needs to be present to achieve the beneficial outcome, Davidson needs to be absent. The problem that needs to be solved is intimately bound up with Davidson, but completely independent of Kolbe. If Kolbe had never existed, the Jewish father would have died. Had Davidson never existed, no medical resources would have been bound up. The same is true of the examples given above. The pilot who stays onboard a burning plane to steer it away from a populated area and the soldier who throws himself onto a grenade need to exist to make the good outcome happen. On the other hand, Captain Oates needs to be absent, as does Gary Davidson, to achieve the desired outcome.

Of course, we ought to note that the comparison between Davidson and Oates only works within a system of limited medical resources where resources freed are indeed making a difference for somebody. In highly affluent countries such as the United States, a situation in which a patient wishes to die in order to free medical resources should—obviously—not arise.

One could therefore argue that self-sacrifice has four rather than three conditions. In addition to the previous conditions, it is an essential part of self-sacrifice that the person involved needs to be present to achieve the good outcome. So patients who give their lives to save medical resources cannot be classed as self-sacrificers, as it is their non-existence that is aimed at (to save medical resources). If this is true, what are people like Nietzsche and Lamm demanding with their "duty to die" claim? If it is not self-sacrifice, is there another distinction that can be made to define such instances satisfactorily? To answer these questions, two new classes of self-caused deaths have to be introduced, both based on anthropological research by Emile Durkheim.

According to Durkheim, "suicide ... is surely very common among primitive peoples. But it displays peculiar characteristics." [23] The peculiar characteristics Durkheim recorded fall into three categories.

- Suicides of men on the brink of old age, or of being seriously ill.
- Suicides of women upon their husbands' death.
- Suicides of followers pursuing their deceased chiefs into death.

Durkheim characterizes the above types of suicide as "obligatory altruistic suicides."[24] Given our definition of altruism (the practice of disinterested and selfless concern for the well-being of others), we could ask whether these suicides are really altruistic. It is not exactly obvious whose well-being is being served when the widow of a recently deceased man is being burnt alive (*suttee*, voluntary widow burning). At least, we could argue that children and other relatives are being subjected to an unnecessary loss at a time when they are already grieving. Likewise we could ask whose well-being is being maximized by the deaths of men closely connected to a chief? Consequently, the word "altruistic" seems unsuitable to characterize these types of suicides.

However, the first group, that of old and ill men choosing death over dependency, falls into a gray area if we limit all considerations to economic usefulness. The men in question could conceivably be viewed to contribute to overall well-being and to act altruistically by wanting to save resources. They could also be regarded as the pre-modern equivalent of the Gary Davidson case. So, I shall look at the specific characteristics of Durkheim's "obligatory altruistic suicides" (OAS) to see whether they conceptually explain those who might follow a "duty to die" as demanded by Lamm.

- The act of suicide is expected from those who commit OAS. Death is imposed by society as a duty on all those in the above-named specific situations (widows, followers, old men). It is a question of honor to acknowledge this duty, or accept loss of public respect.[25]
- OASs are culturally determined. A particular society has to have a particular approach to duty and death in order to command suicides of this nature. In modern Western culture, the widow who kills herself upon her husband's death might be considered egoistic rather than altruistic, at least if she leaves behind children.

- The duties of OASs apply universally to the whole population of one culture (given they come to belong to certain groups), whereas we would not demand universally that humans act like Maximilian Kolbe. So, the duties of OAS are compulsory, whilst the duties of self-sacrifice are supererogatory.
- The duty of OAS applies to specific groups of persons. It has to be the widow who is being burned with her husband, not their children or any other person. The same applies to the Chief's followers and members of the third group (ill and old men).

Based on this brief analysis of the above cases from Durkheim's research, we can make two further classifications to answer the question under consideration (if Gary Davidson is not a self-sacrificer, how could he be classified?). The two categories required are subsets of suicide, namely "altruistic suicide" and "obligatory honorable suicide." An "altruistic suicide" is a suicide characterized by the practice of disinterested and selfless concern for the well-being of others. In contrast to self-sacrifice, however, the person wanting to commit suicide is part of the perceived problem. The second new category, "obligatory honorable suicide," has four main characteristics: suicide is imposed by society as a duty; suicides are culturally regulated; suicides are compulsory, not supererogatory; and suicides are restricted to certain groups. Which cases of physician-assisted self-caused deaths fit our three categories (self-sacrifice, altruistic suicide, obligatory honorable suicide)?

Physician-assisted self-sacrifice: A case of physician-assisted self-sacrifice could be hypothetically constructed as follows. A mother of two twin daughters suffering from kidney failure becomes a live donor to one of her daughters. The kidney transplantation is successful and she demands to have her last kidney removed to benefit her second daughter. She does not wish to die but instead wants to use dialysis to stay alive. Although she survives the operation, complications of which she was aware and which were very likely to occur during her first dialysis lead to her death. This hypothetical case fits all of the requirements for self-sacrifice as outlined above. So, we can answer the first of two main questions set at the outset of this chapter. Is physician-assisted self-sacrifice possible? Yes, it is theoretically possible. However, there rightly are legal restrictions on this type of behavior and so, if it occurs at all, it is extremely rare. The most likely case is probably in pregnancy, when—for instance—an expectant mother refuses chemotherapy for a very aggressive tumor, with the foreseeable result that the baby survives but the mother dies.

Altruistic physician-assisted suicide and *obligatory honorable physician-assisted suicide*: The main distinguishing factor between these two sub-sets of suicide is the content of the main intention involved in the action. Those committing altruistic physician-assisted suicide have a strong intention that is characterized by extraordinarily selfless concern for the well-being of others. They are not self-sacrificers, as their non-existence rather than their existence is essential to achieving the desired outcome. Those committing obligatory honorable physician-assisted suicide strongly intend to fulfill a culturally regulated, compulsory duty imposed by society on certain groups. Gary Davidson could fit both descriptions.

In societies with vastly extended life expectancies coupled with frailness and ill health in old age and serious financial pressures on health systems, thoughts of a "duty to die" can arise, as the examples of Lamm and Hardwig showed. Also, most opponents of physician-assisted suicide and euthanasia argue that these procedures will "lessen our respect for human life and our sense of responsibility for the weak, vulnerable, and infirm."[26] One way to look at this objection is to say that those raising it are trying to stop society from imposing such a duty or from creating the type of coercive setting conducive to demands from Lamm and Hardwig. It is not yet the case that physician-assisted suicide is considered a duty, but it is conceivable in the climate of scarce resources and rationing, as the New York State Task Force on Life and the Law noted when claiming:

> If we allow assisted suicide, then although nominally the request must originate from the patient, physicians will exercise a degree of coercion and/or persuasion that is illegitimate. This is particularly likely in the current context where there is growing concern about increasing health care costs. It will be far less costly to give a lethal injection than to care for a patient throughout the dying process.[27]

Two commentators on the Davidson case remark separately that social pressure might explain his apparent altruism. Sophia Vinogradov and Joe E. Thornton write: "In a period of scarce resources, a vulnerable and distressed patient who is labeled as nonproductive or deviant by society may feel that he does not deserve life-sustaining medical treatment."[28] A. J. Rock Levinson demands that Davidson's doctor seek further consultation with the patient's family, who endorsed his decision to die too easily, in his opinion. He wants to know whether "they are all afraid that Mr Davidson's recovery from this crisis will create for them the burden and threat of caring for an AIDS victim ."[29] Again, the social burden element is strongly apparent in this commentary. We cannot determine Gary Davidson's true intentions. He might have had a genuine and very strong wish to help others by freeing medical resources (altruistic suicide), or he might have been manipulated and coerced into his decision (obligatory honorable suicide). Although this cannot be finally established, we can now answer our second major question set at the outset of this chapter: Is physician-assisted self-sacrifice or its near relatives—altruistic physician-assisted suicide or obligatory honorable physician-assisted suicide—morally desirable?

- Obligatory honorable suicides have a very strong element of coercion and manipulation. Having cultural expectations about death and who counts as a burden is only possible where individuals are sacrificed for social ends. This violates the Kantian principle of never using a person as a means only,[30] a principle widely accepted in rights-based liberal democracies.
- Self-sacrificers and altruistic suicides should be regarded as what they are: exceptional moral heroes. To transfer moral praise from what they have done to obligatory honorable suicide disregards the fact that the former are morally outstanding and incomparable, whilst the latter demands the same conduct from everybody. It thereby tacitly moves from supererogatory acts to compulsory moral duties, a move that cannot be justified.

So, self-sacrifice and altruistic suicide are clear instantiations of morally praiseworthy heroism. Obligatory honorable suicides, on the other hand, can never be normatively endorsed. They are an injustice imposed on the weak.

5. Conclusion

Suicide and self-sacrifice can be distinguished as long as we allow mental concepts to play a role. Suicide can then be defined as death resulting directly or indirectly from a strongly intended positive or negative act of the victim herself, which she knows will produce this result. Self-sacrifice differs from suicide in so far as death is only foreseen but unwanted, whilst the strongly intended part of the action is undertaken out of extraordinarily selfless concern for the well-being of others. In addition, the self-sacrificer's presence is essential to the beneficial outcome that is being aimed at.

Exploring the question "How does self-sacrifice relate to physician-assisted suicide?" three categories were distinguished.

- Physician-assisted self-sacrifice is characterized by a main intention showing extraordinarily selfless concern for others, as well as the non-necessity of one's own death for the desired outcome. Consequently, death is foreseen and wanted.
- Altruistic physician-assisted suicide is identical to self-sacrifice but requires the suicide's death as part of the desired outcome.
- Obligatory honorable physician-assisted suicide is characterized by culturally regulated, compulsory duties imposed by society on certain groups under certain circumstances.

To conclude: it was argued that obligatory honorable suicides must not be imposed on anybody, as this would imply sacrificing individuals for social ends, a practice that is unacceptable in rights-based liberal democracies. Likewise, the heroism of self-sacrifice and altruistic suicide, which is supererogatory, should never be demanded as a compulsory duty from the weak, the vulnerable, and the elderly. There can never be a duty to die.

NOTES

1. Terence O'Keefe, "Suicide and Self-Starvation," *Suicide—Right or Wrong*?, ed. John Donnelly (New York, NY: Prometheus, 2nd ed., 1998), p. 141; Strachan Donnelly, "Views of Human Nature," *The Concise Encyclopaedia of the Ethics of New Technologies*, ed. Ruth Chadwick (San Diego: Academic Press, 2001), p. 20.

2. Gerald Dworkin, "Public Policy and Physician-Assisted Suicide," *Euthanasia and Physician-Assisted Suicide*, ed. Gerald Dworkin, R. G. Frey, and S. Bok (Cambridge: Cambridge University Press, 1998), p. 68.

3. Quoted in Margaret Pabst Battin, *Ethical Issues in Suicide* (Englewood Cliffs: Prentice Hall, 1982), p. 99.

4. Friedrich Nietzsche, "Götzendämmerung," *Jenseits von Gut und Böse und andere Schriften—Werke 3* (Köln: Könemann Verlagsgesellschaft, 1994), p. 357 (my own translation).

5. Pabst Battin, *Ethical Issues in Suicide*, p. 58.

6. John Hardwig, "Is There a Duty to Die?," *Hastings Center Report*, 27:2 (1997), pp. 34–42.

7. Emile Durkheim, *Suicide* (London: Routledge and Kegan Paul, 1952), p. 44.

8. Tom Beauchamp, "Suicide," *Matters of Life and Death*, ed. Tom Regan (New York, NY: McGraw-Hill, 1993), pp. 73f; William Tolhurst, "Suicide, Self-Sacrifice, and Coercion," *Suicide—Right or Wrong?*, ed. Donnelly, pp. 105–117.

9. Durkheim, *Suicide*, pp. 37f.

10. Tolhurst, "Suicide, Self-Sacrifice, and Coercion," p. 107.

11. Beauchamp, "Suicide," pp. 73f.

12. Thomas Aquinas, "The Catholic View," *Suicide—Right or Wrong?*, ed. Donnelly, pp. 40–42; Pabst Battin, *Ethical Issues in Suicide*, pp. 27–63.

13. Tolhurst, "Suicide, Self-Sacrifice, and Coercion," p. 108.

14. Gerald Dworkin, "Introduction," *Euthanasia and Physician-Assisted Suicide*, ed. Gerald Dworkin, R. G. Frey, and S. Bok., p. 3.

15. *Ibid.*

16. R. G. Frey, "Distinctions in Death," *Euthanasia and Physician-Assisted Suicide*, ed. Dworkin *et al*, p. 27.

17. Durkheim, *Suicide*.

18. Beauchamp, "Suicide," p. 109; Dworkin, "Public Policy and Physician-Assisted Suicide," p. 68.

19. Anon., "If I Have AIDS, Then Let Me Die Now!," *Hastings Center Report*, 14:1 (1984), p. 24.

20. *Ibid.*

21. Felicia Cohn and Joanne Lynn, "A Duty to Care," *Is There a Duty to Die?*, ed. John Hardwig (New York/London: Routledge, 2000), p. 145.

22. R. G. Frey, "Distinctions in Death," p. 39.

23. Durkheim, *Suicide*, p. 219.

24. *Ibid.*, p. 221.

25. *Ibid.*, p. 219.

26. Strachan Donnelley, "Views of Human Nature," *The Concise Encyclopedia of the Ethics of New Technologies*, ed. Ruth Chadwick (San Diego: Academic Press, 2001), p. 250.

27. New York State Task Force on Life and the Law, *When Death is Sought: Assisted Suicide and Euthanasia in the Medical Context* (Albany, NY: 1994), p. 123.

28. Sophia Vinogradov and Joe E. Thornton, "Commentary on 'If I Have AIDS, Then Let Me Die Now!,'" *Hastings Center Report*, 14:1 (1984), p. 25.

29. A. J. Rock Levinson, "Commentary on 'If I Have AIDS, Then Let Me Die Now!,'" *Hastings Center Report*, 14:1 (1984), p. 25.

30. Immanuel Kant, *Grundlegung zur Metaphysik der Sitten* (Hamburg: Felix Meiner Verlag, 1965), p. 52.

Three

FORGET AUTONOMY AND GIVE ME FREEDOM!

Matti Häyry

1. The Questions

Suppose that I am in considerable pain. Suppose, further, that I have, by consulting medical literature, become convinced that cannabis is the solution to my problems—that smoking marijuana would alleviate my pain without causing disproportionate side effects. Should I, in this case, be free to use cannabis to make me feel better? And would this be required by respect for my autonomy?

The standard responses link the answers to these questions together. Some say that I should be free to make this choice because it is required by my autonomy, while others contend that I should not be free to do so because it is not in line with my autonomy. But is it necessary to make this connection? I do not think so.

My claim in this chapter is that autonomy can be inimical to freedom: in other words, that respect for the autonomy of persons can lead to disrespect as regards their individual liberty. This is a modestly sensational claim. It is widely assumed in healthcare ethics that the freedom of individuals is best protected by paying heed to the principle of self-determination, or autonomy. But my claim is that this is not the case—or, at least, that this is not always the case. Respect for autonomy can lead to restrictions of freedom.

I will defend my claim by answering four interrelated questions. These are:

- What is freedom?
- Why should freedom be respected?
- What is autonomy?
- Why should autonomy be respected?

After these considerations, I will conclude by reformulating the claim in terms of my example, and by outlining an argument for preferring freedom to autonomy in this and similar cases.

2. What is Freedom?

In this chapter, I take freedom to mean the non-restriction of options. In other words, an individual is free to the degree that her options remain open to her. And, conversely, an individual is unfree to the extent that her options are ruled out by clearly definable constraints—which can be external or internal, positive or negative.

Within this definition, nobody is perfectly free. Due to physical limitations, human beings cannot fly like eagles, swim like sharks, or jump like tigers. Due to economic constraints, most people cannot afford to buy a new car every month, and some people cannot even afford to buy food every day. Due to gaps in education, many people cannot make informed decisions regarding their own lives. And due to social and cultural restrictions, many people cannot express their true opinions without fear of untoward consequences.

Healthcare professionals can respect, and promote, the freedom of their patients in two ways. They can try not to eliminate any options open to the patients before the professional contact. And they can try to remove physical, economic, educational, and social constraints by their professional efforts and by civic participation.

3. Why Should Freedom be Respected?

The answer to my second question can be found in the seventeenth-century liberal doctrine usually attributed to John Locke. According to this doctrine, individuals have rights. The most important of these are:

- the right to life;
- the right to health;
- the right to liberty;
- the right to bodily integrity;
- the right to private property; and
- the right to punish those who violate other people's rights.

These rights are, essentially, entitlements to non-interference. Other people should not actively attempt to end our lives, corrupt our health, steal our property, or curtail our freedom of choice. If they do, or attempt to do, any of these, they partly lose their original entitlements, and we have the right to punish them, or prevent them from wrongdoing by threats of punishment.

The rights individuals possess are, in this model, based on the idea that people do not in the end belong to themselves, but to God. We have a strict duty not to interfere with the lives, health, and liberty of other individuals, because they should be left free to manage their God-given lives for themselves. They should do this in the best way they can, in the light of their reason and understanding. But even if they do not, we cannot legitimately interfere so long as they do not violate the rights of others.

4. What is Autonomy?

The definition of autonomy usually employed in healthcare ethics can be traced back to the eighteenth-century philosophy of Immanuel Kant. He held the view that autonomy means personal self-determination in the light of universal reason. People can, according to his doctrine, be "truly free" only in the realm of rationality. If they yield to their desires, attitudes, or emotions, they reject their autonomy (and their true freedom).

Since desires, attitudes, and emotions are a constant factor in our lives, Kant believed that people cannot be perfectly autonomous. But he argued that we have a moral duty to try to achieve this impossible goal. It follows from this that if other people know better than we what the requirements of universal reason are, then we should not oppose their paternalistic guidance. It is, after all, our own autonomy (or rational self-determination) that is promoted by the intervention.

5. Why Should Autonomy be Respected?

Kant thought that we should celebrate our autonomy, because it is the only thing that can distinguish us from the rest of the world, and make us moral. Desires, attitudes, and emotions belong to the empirical world, which can be encountered only as a predetermined sequence of causes and effects. In this prearranged world of phenomena, there is no freedom of choice, hence no responsibility for one's actions, and hence no morality.

But we yearn to be moral, and we yearn to be a part of another world, the world of things as they really are. In this world of pure thought, freedom and morality are possible, and we must, to be moral, imitate this other world by acting as autonomously as we can.

To reiterate, morality requires freedom, but freedom is not possible in the empirical realm. It is only possible in the rational realm, and hence, to be moral, human beings must strive to be rational. And rationality demands respect for rational self-determination.

6. Practical Implications

My final question is, what would respect for freedom and respect for autonomy imply in the case of prescribing cannabis to alleviate pain, where the patient has expressed a clear preference in its favor?

As regards *freedom*, legislation obviously plays an important role in what health professionals can and cannot do. If the use of marijuana for medical purposes is legally allowed, then health professionals would, by denying a request for it, rule out an existing option, and thereby explicitly restrict their patient's freedom. If, on the other hand, the use of cannabis is prohibited, the option is not in the same way open to patients before the consultation. It can be argued that under these circumstances the freedom of the patient making the request is not actively restricted by the professionals. But since the option remains closed, the freedom of the individual is not maximally promoted, either. (It could be further enhanced by attempts to legalize marijuana.)

This means that, whatever the legal situation, respect for the freedom of the individual would imply that requests like this should be granted, either by health professionals or by society as a whole.

When it comes to autonomy, however, the situation is different. Respect for autonomy can, theoretically speaking, lead to the same norm as respect for freedom. It can be argued that universal reason, if interpreted correctly, would not oppose the use of (even otherwise forbidden) recreational drugs, provided there are good medical grounds for this.

But at least in the original Kantian setting, additional work would be needed to show that this does not go against the categorical imperative—the requirement that moral rules must be equally applicable to all relevantly similar cases. If the point of my example is the reduction of physical pain, then what about extending the rule to cases where everyday mental discomfort or boredom could be relieved by the same method?

The standard Kantian objection at this point would be that the use of cannabis confuses the mind and leads to addiction. These are serious accusations, since both bafflement and chemical dependency can be seen to hinder rational, self-deter-mined decision-making. And, in the name of consistency, it seems that these accus-ations must be extended to the medical use of marijuana, lest people start to think that it would be all right to confuse one's mind for purely recreational reasons as well.

This is why respect for autonomy in the Kantian sense would support restrictions more probably than freedom. And this is what I set out to prove in this paper: *that respect for autonomy can lead to restrictions of freedom.*

7. Autonomy or Freedom?

Let me conclude by presenting the possible combinations of respect and disrespect for the two principles, and by stating my own preference among them.

There are, from the purely conceptual point of view, four alternatives, which are presented schematically in the following table:

	Disrespect for Freedom	Respect for Freedom
Respect for Autonomy	(1) Universal reason demands that we restrict freedom when this is needed to protect rational self-determination.	(2) Universal reason reveals that freedom and rational self-determ-ination are mutually compatible.
Disrespect For Autonomy	(3) There is no universal reason in ethics, and individual liberty is a secondary consideration.	(4) There is no universal reason that could override the reasons individuals have for their choices.

Alternatives (1) and (2) are open to those who buy into the Kantian notion of autonomy, and they are both feasible responses, although in the case of prescribing cannabis the formulation of (2) can be difficult. Alternative (3) could represent a traditional, or communitarian, response, where prevailing attitudes and their conformity to the values of the society in question would be paramount. Alternative (4) is my own favorite. It is an ultra-liberal view, which rejects even “rational self-determination” because of the potential paternalism implicit in the Kantian view.

One way to defend the ultra-liberal view would be to follow Locke, and to say that no one should interfere with the individual liberty given to us by God. This defense does not necessarily summon any particular view of God, religion, or theology. It can be taken simply to mean that our individuality is an extremely valuable thing, and that attempts, by others, to mess with it cannot add anything to its value. To use a metaphor popular in bioethical debates, we could say that others are trying to “play God” if they claim that their rationality should override our choices.

It remains to be added that even within the ultra-liberal view, restrictions of liberty can be justified, and attempts to promote the rational self-determination of others can be legitimate. Restrictions of liberty are justified, if freely chosen actions would inflict harm on others. And those who think that recreational drugs diminish the autonomy of persons, can, of course, make their views known, and try to persuade others to share them.

But until somebody gives me good grounds for thinking otherwise, my view in this and in similar cases is: *Forget autonomy and give me freedom!*

8. Discussion

This paper was presented in the Fifth International Bioethics Retreat in Almagro, Spain, 3–9 June 2002. In the ensuing discussion, the following questions were asked. I wrote them down some time after the session, and I apologize for any inaccuracies. My answers below are based on my original responses, but may be slightly idealized, or enhanced, since I have had time to think about them following the Retreat.

Sharon Sytsma: "Pain can reduce autonomy so that removing the pain, even by confusing and addictive substances, would be acceptable on Kantian grounds."

MH: Point taken, but is there ever autonomy in the Kantian sense in these situations? If you are in pain, you are not autonomous. But if the pain is taken away with confusing drugs, you will be confused, and hence not autonomous, either.

Jan Hartman: "The traditional thick concept of freedom can accommodate the distinction between real and illusory freedom. This is an important distinction. Can the thin concept of freedom you use in your paper accommodate it?"

MH: Yes, I think it can. John Locke makes the distinction between being free and feeling free in *An Essay Concerning Human Understanding* (Vol. I: II, xxi, 10), where he cites the case of a man who voluntarily stays in a room chatting with a long lost friend but is actually unfree because the door is locked.

Zbigniew Zalewski: "Saying that the justification of liberty is that it is *my* liberty means committing the naturalistic fallacy."

Griffin Trotter: "Well, yes, but saying that it does means committing the rationalistic or universalistic fallacy."

Rosamond Rhodes: Harry Frankfurt distinguishes between first and second order desires. I can have a desire to eat cookies but also a desire not to have a desire to eat cookies. With regard to which of these must freedom be restricted?

MH: Whichever *you* choose. But it is against my freedom if somebody else decides to restrict the fulfillment of my "first order" desires in the name of my "second order" (or "higher" or "more rational") desires.

Constance Perry: "But what should be done, if a person high on crack does not want any treatment, even if the medics know that it would be vital?"

MH: It is possible within the ultra-liberal view to draw a distinction between occurrent confusion and permanent addiction. If a person is temporarily confused, the medics can sometimes legitimately administer treatments against the patient's wishes. But if people permanently addicted to drugs do not want to be "cured" from this condition, let them be (unless they inflict harm on others).

Four

CHOOSING BETWEEN CLAIMS: ALLOCATING PARENTAL RESPONSIBILITY IN SURROGACY DISPUTES

Monique Jonas

1. Introduction

If King Solomon was faced with a perplexing dilemma when called upon to establish which of two women's claims to motherhood was genuine, then surely our modern day Solomons, Dame Elizabeth Butler-Sloss and the British Human Fertilization and Embryology Authority amongst them, have predicaments of the first order to contend with. Some of the contemporary dilemmas over parental rights are due to the fact that today's reproductive environment is characterized by so much new possibility: it is now possible, for instance, for five distinct individuals to make essential contributions to one conception and pregnancy (a genetic mother, a genetic father, a gestating mother, and a commissioning couple), or for a person to become a genetic parent entirely unawares and with someone they have never met (through the mistaken use of their genetic material in an IVF pregnancy). When understandings about pregnancies or allocation of parental responsibility break down, or mistakes happen at conception, the means by which to resolve ensuing disputes are not at all clear.

Although the technology involved here is new and some of the dilemmas arising from its use take new forms, their content is as old as Solomon himself. The desire to raise a child is something that many people feel very strongly, and parenthood imbues many lives with a sense of profound meaning. So when more than one couple identify a given child as their "own," the conflict that follows is likely to reflect this sense of personal import. Conflicts over parental rights, and, more specifically, the need to resolve them, give us the opportunity, and indeed the necessity, to examine what it is that we consider important about parenthood, and what purpose we want parental responsibility to serve.

In this chapter, I propose to consider three factors that are relevant to the resolution of disputes over parental responsibility: genetic contribution, labor, and contracts or promises. Ordinarily, in our society, one couple or family group provides all the contributions necessary to procreation, but in surrogacy disputes and other conflicts over parental responsibility, genetic and labor-based contributions can be split across several different parties, and contracts regarding the care of the child may exist. How much significance each of these factors ought to be accorded is by no means clear, but by considering what it is that we value about these three things, I hope to cast light upon the respective roles that they should play in the resolution of parental rights conflicts.

In order to consider the relative weight of different kinds of parental responsibility claim in isolation, I am going to assume that the parties competing for parental responsibility are each able to provide for (at least) the basic interests of the child in question (however those basic interests come to be defined). Where one party is clearly not able to secure the child's basic interests, there is an argument for placing the child with the party that can do so, even if the first party has the stronger claim, independently of those interests. Although the strength of a claim to parental responsibility need not be divorced from considerations of the child's interests, other factors might be at play too, and by removing concerns for the child, I hope to get at those factors.

For the purposes of this chapter, I will use the terms "parental rights" and "parental responsibility" interchangeably, on the assumption that people seek legal status as a person with parental responsibility primarily to attain the rights conferred thereby (especially the rights to cohabit with and be the primary care-taker of and decision-maker for the child).[1] Although I will focus here on conflicts arising from surrogacy agreements, I contend that my central claims will hold true for other kinds of parental rights disputes, too.

2. Genetic Contributions

Genetics plays a major role in the allocation of parental rights, a role that pre-dates the entry of the concept of genetics into the common imagination. The people who make direct genetic contributions to the conception of a child are thought of as her parents, at least in the first instance, and have first option on the assumption of parental responsibility. Society recognizes a right to rear those persons whom one bears, and this right is revoked in only the most extreme of circumstances. Ordinarily, this distribution of rights and responsibilities works pretty well; generally the people responsible for conceiving a child are more willing to invest the time and resources in her upbringing than anybody else, so the practice is a happy one. In common or garden conceptions, there is no need to determine whether custody is being awarded on the basis of genetics, or labor, or the undertakings of a contract: there is no conflict based on these disparate contributions to preside over. But in those instances in which these contributions do come into conflict (and such instances may well multiply as a result of reproductive technology), the rationale for the presumption in favor of genetics is tested. So, what is it about genetic parenthood that is so important: why does the genetic relationship between parent and child ground a claim to parental rights?

One explanation for the unique privileges that biological parents have with regard to their children is that children are the property of their parents: just as I own my arms and legs, or, more controversially, my genetic information, so I own the children that issue from me. There is something very uncomfortable about this notion: to accept it would be to accept that every child is born into a kind of slavery. But if one accepts certain prominent theories of property ownership, then it is difficult to avoid accepting this approach to parental rights as well.[2]

And there are good reasons to avoid accepting this view of parental rights. The relationship between an owner and the thing she owns is one characterized by rights rather than responsibilities. If I own a car, the rights that I have over it are not conditional upon my taking care of it: I can smother it with oil and adoration, leave it to slowly rust into oblivion, or strip its innards and transplant them into another car according to my merest whim. We do not think that we owe anything to the things that we own (although there are some possible exceptions to this, pets and English listed property amongst them), but we do think that parents owe their children certain things and consider that treatment of children should be governed by more than parental whim. Instead, it should be governed by a respect for, and desire to protect, their well-being. Ownership does not seem to encapsulate the subtle weave of rights and responsibilities that tie parents and children together.

But the objection that genetic parenthood cannot ground a claim to parental ownership does not rob the genetic relationship of all its possibility here. One could accept that genetic parenthood is not akin to ownership (perhaps because children are not the sort of things that can legitimately be owned) and still accept that whatever parental rights there are derive from the existence of a genetic relationship. What kinds of claims could substantiate this assertion?

One way of justifying the extension of parental rights on the grounds of genetic relationships is by appealing to the essential nature of that contribution. If it were not for the fact that x and y contributed their genetic information, z would never have existed.[3] In other cases in which a person (or group of persons) has made all the contributions required to create something, we think that this fact is enough to warrant the extension of special rights to the creator with regard to the thing created. This kind of rights-extension need not be based upon any positive claim about the nature of creation; it might instead be justified by a negative assertion that nobody else has a better claim, and in the absence of something better, the creator's claim stands.

This is plausible, but problematic. In the case of children, although genetic contribution is essential, it is not the only essential thing. A favorable environment for gestation, and, in the case of problematic conceptions and pregnancies, the assistance of expert medical staff, can also be essential to the creation of a new life. How are we to differentiate between the contributions made by a genetic father, that of an obstetrician whose treatment is essential to the safe delivery of a troublesome pregnancy, and the skilful labor of the medical technician who performs the in vitro fertilization (IVF) procedure that facilitates conception? Without the contribution of each, the child would not have been born; in that sense, each contribution was essential. If we want to avoid the extension of parental responsibility to hard-working obstetricians and IVF clinicians, we will have to explain what kinds of essential contribution count here, and why.

It might be possible to do this by distinguishing between identity-affecting contributions (and the claims that they can support) and non-identity affecting contributions. An obstetrician or reproductive scientist might have furnished the help essential to the child's life, but whilst those contributions were essential to the creation of the baby, neither had an effect on the identity of that baby. The child would have been the same child regardless of who delivered it or who injected the ova with sperm. The child would not have had the same identity, however, if its genetic material had been derived from different people than it in fact was.

Another way to express this might involve a distinction between creation on the one hand and nurture or support on the other: one could accept that a child's conception and birth can rely upon the support of people other than the genetic parents, but claim that that support is fundamentally different from the contribution entailed by actual creation.

Whilst efforts such as these may be capable of bearing theoretical fruit, I suspect that they will prove to be both riddled with problems and importantly beside the point. There might be differences between identity-affecting creation and essential contributions of support, but how much moral weight can such distinctions bear, and what difference do they make to rights allocation (note how the distinction looks set to break down in the case of the IVF technician, handpicking the sperm used to fertilize ova)? It is likely that the process of establishing what identity-affecting creation actually entails (and excludes) would be so problematic as to be worth avoiding.

I think that there is another, simpler way to identify what is valuable about genetic parenthood. Genetic parents tend to care deeply about their genetic offspring, and identify their interests as being tied up with their children's welfare in a way that they are not with other children (even other children with whom they share a "blood" relation, such as nieces and cousins). This strong identification means that genetic parents profit more, in general, from the extension of parental responsibility than other people would, and that they have more to lose than anyone else if parental rights are denied or revoked.

There are also important spin-off effects for the children raised by their genetic parents. Because, in general, people identify a greater personal interest in their "own" genetic children than others, they are more likely to want the best for their children, and will more easily make personal sacrifices to secure their children's interests, than other people are likely to. Thus, both genetic parents, and their progeny, generally profit from the allocation of parental responsibility on this basis. So, there are strong consequentialist reasons to support a general presumption in favor of awarding genetic parents parental responsibility.

One of the features of consequentialist justifications is that they can only really function as justifications for given policies or acts if those policies or acts do, in fact, bring about the intended ends (maximization of the preferred good). So, extension of parental rights to genetic parents is only supported by the above claims in those cases in which three conditions hold:

- genetic parents really do have deep and abiding interests in assuming parental responsibility;
- those interests lead them to strive for their children's interests; and
- no other party has deeper or more abiding interests tied up with those children.

In most instances, these three conditions hold true, and the vast majority of cases in which they do not are very likely (in contexts other than surrogacy conflicts and the like) to be cases in which removing children from their genetic parents would be an acceptable option (because the children are being neglected or abused, or because their basic interests are not able to be secured within their family home). In these cases, the link is broken between genetic parenthood and its use as a justification for parental rights extension by a failure to meet one or both of the first two conditions (that is, the genetic parents do not have abiding interests in their children's well-being or that those interests, whilst present, do not lead them to strive for their children's interests). Thus, the allocation of parental responsibility on the basis of genetic parenthood fails to perform its function and other solutions must be looked to. The consequentialist approach to parental rights attributes a qualified importance to genetic parenthood: a general assumption in favor of the genetic parents is justified, but if, in a given case, the genetic parents do not in fact fulfill their obligations or develop an attachment to their child, that assumption is able to be overridden.

The central problem with this justification in the context of failed surrogacy arrangements does not arise because one or both of the first two conditions is not met, but because the third does not hold true. Here, the genetic parents are generally not the only parties with deep and abiding interests in the assumption of parental responsibility—the dispute arises precisely because there are other parties who identify a fundamental interest in raising the child in question, are willing to strive for the child's well-being, and earnestly seek assumption of parental responsibility. The reasons that we care about genetic parenthood in general also apply to people other than the genetic parents and so, in these cases, genetic parenthood does not provide the solid ground for parental rights claims that it does in common or garden conceptions—it becomes just one claim among several. Because the surrogate mother with no genetic relationship to the baby she carried, or the commissioning mother, or the father whose partner carried "someone else's baby" through an IVF mix-up, could want and care for the child just as much as those people with verifiable genetic relationships with her, the claim from genetics loses some (but not all) of its power.

So, with regard to surrogacy disputes and other conflicts over parental rights, the genetic contribution grounds a claim worthy of consideration, but it is not a lone contender. The force of the genetic claim, in my account, lies in the fact that people care more, as a rule, about children that they identify as their own, and identify strong interests in raising them as such. In surrogacy disputes, parties other than genetic parents may come to the table with these self-same reasons for lodging a parental rights claim, so resolution will require the consideration of other factors. This explanation of the importance of the genetic relationship offers no quick fixes in conflicts like those under consideration here, but it goes some way to explaining why disputes of the kind that failed surrogacy agreements give rise to, are so complex. Examination of the case to be made for labor and contracts will cast light upon ways in which resolution may be sought.

3. Labor

A claim very like the one considered above for genetics can be made on the basis of labor. There are two kinds of labor, or more accurately, periods of labor, that would be of relevance when judging claims to parental responsibility. The first is labor invested before birth, the second is labor invested afterwards. Because disputes that spring from surrogacy-related conflicts are likely to happen while the child in question is in infancy, and because conflicts that occur later would be smattered with other considerations (such as the parental relationships that the child is likely to have developed), I wish to concentrate on pre-birth labor. We can assume that the candidates for parental responsibility will be equally willing to labor for the benefit of the child after birth, given that we have specified that the child will enjoy an equally good upbringing in either home. So, the labor invested prior to the conflict will be considered here.

Perhaps the most interesting kind of labor that takes place before birth is that which a gestating mother performs in relation to the fetus she carries, although the claim that gestation involves labor is not without controversy. It can be held that the processes involved in, and energy expended upon, the support of a fetus do not constitute labor, or at least not the kind of labor that we would want to attribute to the gestating woman. The claim here is that, although a woman may choose to continue with her pregnancy, and thereby elect to support a fetus, the actual process of support is largely out of her control—her body performs the necessary functions without any conscious instruction from her, and without her being aware that those functions are even taking place. Saying that a woman has "labored" to support her fetus is like saying that I have labored because my liver has performed essential functions necessary to sustain my life. We do not think that the energy and "work," for want of a better word, that the liver expends constitutes labor, or if it does, then it is not the kind of labor that seems intuitively attributable to the individual, as opposed to the individual's liver.

Without wishing to become embroiled in a debate about the requirements necessary for an act to constitute labor, I will claim that an argument can be made for gestation as labor, especially in the case of IVF and surrogacy pregnancies. One of the factors that might be thought to separate labor from other kinds of acts is intention. Other acts that qualify as labor: intellectual labor and physical labor of the stool-making or fruit-picking variety, for instance, differ drastically in their natures, but perhaps one of the qualities that unites them under the labor umbrella is that they are all characterized, and indeed motivated, by intent to work towards some valued ends (this is why we can distinguish between an eminent scientist who spends a career working towards a discovery, and an idle schoolboy who makes a similar discovery while messing about in the school lab). Although those rare pregnancies that take place entirely unbeknownst to the gestating woman would fail to meet this criterion, and so might not qualify as labor (and this could have troubling implications), IVF and surrogacy pregnancies certainly would. In these cases, the gestating women intend their bodies to perform the functions necessary to nurture and sustain fetuses, and go to some considerable lengths to ensure that this happens. On these grounds, and acknowledging the possibility of mounting a serious challenge to them, I want to include gestation in the kinds of labor that might be relevant here.

As in the case of genetics, one of the reasons for thinking that a rights-claim can be advanced on the basis of labor would relate to the essential nature of that labor to the creation of the object in question. Gestational labor certainly qualifies as an essential contribution. But the same problems that hampered this approach with regard to genetics resurface here. And the same simple consequentialist reasons that genetic relationships can be thought to ground rights claims strike me as applicable here too. People tend to care about the things that they create more than other people do, and benefit from recognition of their labor through the extension of rights. This certainly seems to be the case where children are concerned. Surrogate mothers, who did not (initially, at least) intend to rear the children that they bear, often develop strong emotional ties through the process of gestation, and find themselves identifying with the fetus as though it were "theirs." This can happen even when the surrogate is not the genetic mother of the child. After birth, many parents (perhaps especially fathers, who cannot experience the intimacy of gestation in the same way that mothers can) find that their sense of identification with their child deepens, partly as a result of the work involved in looking after them. The investment that labor creates also has benefits for the child: the identification and love that labor can produce in parents in turn generates a willingness to continue working to ensure that the child's needs are met.

Ordinarily, a genetic relationship grounds a willingness to labor, which in turn deepens the commitment to the child. But when genetic contributions and labor are divided between disparate parties, commitments can develop independently and, when disputes occur, oppositionally. So, since both labor and genetic contributions can ground parental responsibility, and because of what amounts to the same reason, how ought our twenty-first century Solomons to negotiate between claims?

4. Contracts and Promises

So far I have identified one reason to acknowledge parental rights (because people identify themselves as having a fundamental interest in their assumption), and two pegs on which that reason may hang (genetic relationships and labor). When two parties present opposing claims to parental responsibility, one on the grounds of a genetic relationship with the child and one on the grounds of the labor that they have so far invested, and if we judge that both claims are of equal importance to the claimants, then it seems as if there is little to choose between them. Some other consideration needs to be introduced as an arbiter, and I wish to consider the case for contract to assume that role.

Surrogacy agreements involve a kind of contract between the gestating woman and the intended parents. This is an aspect of surrogacy that many find objectionable—the prospect of something as intimate as the process of conception, pregnancy, and childbirth being nudged into the realm of trade and contract seems like the ultimate misinterpretation of motherhood and the final victory for "masculine" market values. There appears to be little room in the self-interest drenched world of free trade for appreciation of the emotional content of childbearing. Barbara Katz Rothman is one theorist who expresses these fears. She notes that the language of capitalism has been imported into our vocabulary for the creation of life: "'reproduction,' a word that implies that making babies is a form of production—raw material transformed by work into a product."[4] She also contrasts the "natural" process of gestation with the free market values that taint surrogacy.[5] For Rothman and many others,[6] surrogacy misrepresents the experience of childbearing, takes advantage of women in compromised circumstances in a morally unacceptable fashion, and inappropriately commodifies children by making them the subject of a contract and financial exchange.

It is to be expected that theorists who hold these objections regard the contracts that govern surrogacy arrangements to be of slight moral standing, and maintain that they can never justify the separation of a (birth) mother and her child. It is not my wish to challenge the morality or expediency of surrogacy arrangements, nor am I able to mount an outright defense of the practice here. Suffice it to say that, for the purposes of this discussion, I will hold that agreements between a commissioning party and a prospective gestating mother can amount to ethically (if not legally), valid contracts, although there might be reasons to override those contracts in certain circumstances. I will take it as given that if the surrogate, or the commissioning party for that matter, were misled, insufficiently informed, or less than wholly consenting at the time that the surrogacy agreement was made, this would invalidate the contract. But where an agreement was reached between competent, informed, and consenting individuals to take part in a surrogate pregnancy, I consider that this agreement has moral bearing.

The contract or promise is no stranger to moral theory. Generally speaking, we consider that if we make a promise to someone, we are under a consequent obligation to keep, or at least to take all reasonable steps to keep, the promise that we made. This obligation might be defeasible: some other, more powerful, and conflicting obligation might present itself which trumps the obligation created by the promise, or the promisee might release us from the obligation, or circumstances might change in such a way that the promise is invalidated or notably weakened.[7] But, in the absence of such factors, promises create obligations and constrict our choices.

The question to be addressed here is whether the promises made in surrogacy agreements are defeasible, and if so, what would serve to defeat them? The most commonly espoused justification for the breaking of surrogacy-related promises relates to the unexpected bonding between the gestating mother and her child. The thought here is that the surrogate went into the agreement with false beliefs about how easy it would be to preserve an emotional distance between herself and her pregnancy, and that she could never have anticipated (or, have been reasonably expected to anticipate) the motherly feelings that she would develop for the baby she carried. Whilst she went into the agreement with a sincere commitment to honor it, the reality of the surrogate experience prevented her from being able to realize that commitment, and this constitutes valid grounds for release from the contract.

I find these claims problematic. Entering a surrogacy agreement is an extremely serious step, involving the creation of a child, the deep expectations of others, and what contract law refers to as "reliance interests" in other parties to the contract.[8] In such agreements it is reasonable to expect the parties involved to seriously consider their participation beforehand, and only to make a commitment to the process if they regard it as a commitment that they can honor. Because of the level of seriousness involved, that commitment should be taken as binding on the individuals concerned, and the intentions that characterized their decision to participate, and the reliance that developed upon expression of those intentions, should be taken into consideration if that commitment falters.

There are two considerations that support enforcement of surrogacy contracts, and the first incorporates wider social considerations. Contracts and promises lose their utility if they can be broken because one party has changed their mind, or their situation, or no longer feels committed to the agreed outcome: the assurance that they provide, which enables cooperative activity and all the benefits that accompany it, disappears. So, there are wider social reasons that support the enforcement of contracts, even when enforcement comes at some cost to the promisor. If we decide that gestation is the sort of thing that can be subject to contract, it ought to be subject to the rules of contract.

There is also a more localized reason to adhere, and to enforce adherence, to the contract, and which incorporates considerations of fairness. The surrogate's agreement to gestate a child for the commissioning couple to raise generates both expectations and, I contend, reliance on their part. They prepare themselves for parenthood, the male often makes a genetic contribution (as might the female commissioner), and place their hopes for a family in the agreement: hopes that are likely to have gone unmet to this point, as surrogacy is seldom anyone's first procreative choice. The creation of reliance interests also involves the cutting off of other options: had the surrogate not agreed to perform gestation on their behalf, they may have secured the services of another prospective surrogate, who would have been willing to fulfill the contract. It seems to me that where expectations are the reasonable consequence of the promisor's actions or agreements, the promisor must take some responsibility for them, and that this is best assumed by fulfillment of the contract.

So, for reasons of social utility, as well as fairness, the binding nature of contracts should be preserved, and participants encouraged to consider their participation with the utmost seriousness before committing to them. Having said that, there are certain instances in which it is right to release people from their promises and commitments on the grounds that they have proved more demanding than could reasonably have been anticipated at the time they were made. For instance, I would not hold my friend blameworthy for failing to meet me for coffee when I discover that her car was stolen, leaving her with no transport, and an urgent need to report her vehicle stolen. She had made a commitment that she had every reason to believe she could fulfill, but an unforeseeable event occurred which prevented its fulfillment. Her intentions were good, but events overtook her and her failure to keep her promise does not attract blame.

But there are other instances in which it could be said that difficulties with the keeping of a promise or commitment should have been foreseen and taken into account by its maker. When certain difficulties are very likely to occur, such as would feasibly threaten an agent's ability to honor a commitment, then they should be taken into account by the agent, and if she makes the commitment and then defaults on it, citing these foreseeable difficulties, then she might be held responsible for her failure. For instance, if John promises Sally that he will pick her up after work on Tuesday afternoon, but he knows that he is unlikely to get his car back from the mechanics until Thursday, then Sally would be justified in holding him responsible for his failure to take into account the foreseeable hurdle that lay between him and the keeping of his promise. He knew that it was likely that he would be without transport on Tuesday, but he still made a commitment that hinged upon him having transport then, and so he let Sally down when he was prevented from keeping his promise. It might not be John's fault that his car isn't ready to pick up then, but that doesn't absolve him from all responsibility.

The same might be said of surrogacy cases. It is foreseeable that a surrogate mother will form an emotional bond with the fetus she carries, and that she might have difficulties in surrendering the child when the time comes. This likelihood should be something that the prospective mother considers very seriously before entering into a surrogacy agreement, and if she has any doubts about her ability to adhere to such an agreement, then she should not make it. If she does come to an agreement with a commissioning couple and then finds that she cannot keep it, she might legitimately be accused of failing to take the agreement seriously enough, or of failing to accord enough weight to the possibility that she would become emotionally attached to the baby.

She might reply by saying that, although she knew that it was likely that some women, or even most women, would become thus attached, she could not predict that this would happen to her, because her assessment of her personality and priorities led her to believe that she could remain emotionally unattached. She could not predict what her reaction would be in the way that John could reasonably predict that he would be without transport on Tuesday, because he has concrete information to work with (what the mechanic has told him), while she has only psychological and emotional estimates to make.

There is something in this. We often react to events in ways that we could never have predicted, and in ways that defy our sense of ourselves, and the difficulties with these kinds of predictions warrant consideration, not only by us as assessors after the fact, but also by prospective surrogates (and the people commissioning them). Prospective surrogates should factor into their considerations the chance that their predictions of their reactions to surrogate pregnancy might prove mistaken, and should only enter into such agreement if they can be very sure that they will be able to honor it. If that certainty proves mistaken, we need not attribute blame for such an understandable error to the surrogate, but the contract should be upheld.

It is my view that the fact that circumstances change, and make the keeping of promises more difficult or costly that once anticipated does not absolve a promise-maker or contractor of her voluntarily assumed obligations. Where fate intervenes in a completely unpredictable way, and interferes with an individual's promise-keeping, this ought to be taken into account, and might justify release from the promise. But where the promisor's inclinations simply change, or he develops a preference for not adhering to his contract (and where he might reasonably be expected to have taken this possibility into account), this doesn't constitute grounds for release. So, one important question that bears upon the role of the contract here is whether a surrogate mother can reasonably be expected to anticipate her emotional response to the pregnancy. Some women are able to see themselves as landladies or pre-natal nannies rather than mothers when gestating, and others simply are not.[9] It strikes me that it is up to the prospective surrogate to accurately predict which category she would fit into, and she should be held to her contract if her prediction proves to be mistaken.

5. Conclusion

In a parental rights dispute of this kind, someone always comes out the loser: primary parental responsibility can only be awarded to one household, and that means that at least one claimant will lose one of the things they hold most precious: the chance of forging a traditional parental relationship with a child. In the hardest cases, the stakes are high for all parties, but we have to make a decision in somebody's favor, and I have sketched a method by which this might fairly be done.

According to my analysis, genetic and labor-based contributions both provide grounds for a parental responsibility claim because contributions of those kinds predispose the makers of them to care about the product of their efforts. When labor and genetic contributions to the conception and birth of a child are made by diverse parties, as in surrogacy arrangements, they can come to ground opposing claims. Because they count for the same reason, a third consideration is required to break the tie. I hold that the contract that cements a surrogacy agreement should play that part.

The surrogate's promise to the commissioners created serious reliance interests on their part: they prepared themselves for parenthood because of what she undertook to do for them. If the contract is not honored, these are losses that the surrogate is responsible for; whilst the commissioning party is not responsible for the surrogate's loss in the same way if the contract is enforced, because they never led her to believe that things would be any different. Where surrogacy agreements, which were made on the basis of informed consent, break down, fair resolution will generally involve upholding the contract and according parental responsibility to the commissioning party.

NOTES

1. *Children Act* 1989, section 3.

2. See for instance John Locke, Se*cond Treatise of Government* (Indianapolis, IN: Hackett Publishing, 1980), chapters 5 and 6; John Locke, *Two Treatises of Government*, ed. Peter Laslett (Cambridge: Cambridge University Press, 1967), First Treatise, sections 52–54.

3. See Derek Parfit, *Reasons and Persons* (Oxford: Clarendon Press, 1984).

4. Barbara Katz Rothman, "Recreating Motherhood: Ideology and Technology in American Society," *Beyond Baby M: Ethical Issues in New Reproductive Technologies*, ed. Dianne M. Bartels, Reinhard Priester, Dorothy E. Vawter, and Arthur L. Caplan (Clifton, NJ: Humana Press, 1990).

5. Barbara Katz Rothman, "Surrogacy: A Question of Values," *Beyond Baby M*, ed. Bartels *et al.*

6. See, e.g., Elizabeth Anderson, *Values in Ethics and Economics* (Cambridge, MS: Harvard University Press, 1993); Gena Corea, The Mother Machine (New York, NY: Harper and Row, 1985); Vanessa E. Munro, "Surrogacy and the Construction of the Maternal-Foetal Relationship—the Feminist Dilemma Examined," *Res Publica*, 7:1 (2001), pp. 13–37; Liezl van Zyl and Anton van Niekerk, "Interpretations, Perspectives, and Intentions in Surrogate Motherhood," *Journal of Medical Ethics*, 26:5 (October 2000), pp. 404–410.

7. W. D. Ross, *Foundations of Ethics* (New York, NY: Oxford University Press, 1939), p. 9; Toni Vogel Carey, "How to Confuse Commitment with Obligation," *Journal of Philosophy*, 72:10 (1975), pp. 276–284; Holly Smith, "A Paradox of Promising," *Philosophical Review*, 106:2 (April 1997), pp. 153–196.

8. Gillian Hadfield, "An Expressive Theory of Contract: From Feminist Dilemmas to a Reconceptualization of Rational Choice in Contract Law," *University of Pennsylvania Law Review*, 146:5 (June 1998), pp. 5235–5286.

9. Helena Ragone, *Surrogate Motherhood: Conception in the Heart* (San Francisco, CA: Westview Press, 1994) pp. 75–78; van Zyl and van Niekerk, "Interpretations, Perspectives, and Intentions in Surrogate Motherhood."

Five

THE MANY WRONGS OF HUMAN REPRODUCTIVE CLONING

Tuija Takala

1. Cloning, an Absolute Wrong?

After the birth of the first ever cloned mammal, Dolly the sheep, made the headlines, people all around the world rushed to condemn human cloning as an absolute wrong.[1] A number of laws and treaties were also quickly drafted in this spirit.[2] Subsequent discussions in public, political, and academic fora echoed the denunciation of human cloning, although people were finding it difficult to put their fingers on the exact features that made cloning an absolute wrong. At the same time, however, there were voices excited about the possibilities that cloning humans might create.

In this chapter I will study the main arguments presented against human reproductive cloning. I will start with the most often used counterarguments, namely the arguments from "dignity," "uniqueness," and "treating people as means." After these I will deal briefly with the safety and cost issues. I will show that all the mentioned counterarguments are insufficient to support a total ban on human reproductive cloning. It might be, though, that research ethics will prevent research into human reproductive cloning and, thus, effectively preclude most actual attempts to clone humans. It is further shown that the arguments in favor of cloning are not particularly strong either. The "clone's perspective" on the matter is studied under the claims that cloning is wrong, because it creates "a life in the shadow,"[3] and that it violates the (alleged) "right not to know."

I will show that by employing philosophical methods and arguments, it seems to be impossible to say that there is something absolutely, or *per se*, wrong about human reproductive cloning, although it includes practices that are wrong . By showing in which circumstances cloning is more wrong than in others, these practices are further specified. It is also recognized that the weakness of the arguments in favor of human cloning, and the wrongs (albeit contingent) related to the practice should lead us to conclude that there are no good reasons for investing public money or effort in human reproductive cloning. But we should also conclude that we do not have sufficient reasons to ban human reproductive cloning altogether, if the outstanding safety issues can be properly addressed.

2. What is Cloning?

In discussions on the matter a distinction is usually drawn between therapeutic and reproductive cloning. In the therapeutic variety, the aim is to clone cells that make particular organs or types of tissue, but not entire human beings. While this type of cloning has also been perceived as ethically problematic, it is far better tolerated than the idea of producing new human beings by similar methods (with the perhaps surprising exception of the Catholic Church, which seems to see more problems in therapeutic cloning).[4] In what follows I will deal mainly with issues related to reproductive cloning, and mention the therapeutic alternative only when the arguments used in the debates form a close connection between the two practices.

There are roughly two ways of cloning mammals known to us. The less controversial is "embryo splitting." This happens naturally when one embryo is divided into two or more, thus creating identical twins or, sometimes, triplets or even more. In its artificial form the method has been used with human embryos since 1993.[5] The technique that has raised more moral outrage is the possibility of creating clones by nuclear transfer. This is how Dolly was produced. In this method the nucleus of a cell from another being (in Dolly's case a cell of an adult sheep) is transferred into an unfertilized egg taken from a donor, by a process know as cell fusion.[6] I will concentrate on this more controversial option, although some of the ethical issues overlap with those raised by "embryo splitting." Cloning by nuclear transfer makes possible the creation of a near-identical genetic copy of an existing individual. The closest match can be achieved when the egg and the nucleus come from the same individual. And even when they do not, only residual mitochondrial DNA has its origin in the egg, while all the other genetic material is derived from the transferred nucleus.

3. Is Cloning Humans Against Human Dignity?

Many international protocols and treaties condemn human (reproductive) cloning as an act against human dignity.[7] It is, however, uncertain what exactly human dignity is and why it is violated by human reproductive cloning.[8] As an example of how far apart different understandings of human dignity in relation to cloning are, consider the following quotations.

> The dignity and legal rights of a clone could be guaranteed by a statute ....[9]

> On principle, to replicate any human by technological means is against the basic dignity of the uniqueness of each human being in God's sight.[10]

In the former quotation, dignity seems to be something that is given to humans by humans, while in the latter, our dignity could be interpreted to lie in God's perception of us. In philosophical literature, arguments drawing from human dignity are usually inseparable from arguments employing the ideas that uniqueness has special value and that we should not treat people as a mere means. I will return to these in the following sections.

It seems that the argument from human dignity is used independently only in the contexts of religious ethics and official documents. Not surprisingly, however, even the Christian Church is divided on the question of who is a bearer of human dignity and what this should imply in terms of cloning. As far as the Catholic Church is concerned, any human "material" possesses human dignity in one way or another. Therefore, the Vatican's view on cloning is that therapeutic cloning is at least as bad as (and depending on the interpretation perhaps even worse than) reproductive cloning. This is because therapeutic cloning

> would involve experimentation on embryos and fetuses [a "human being," although in the embryonic state] and would require their suppression before birth—a cruel, exploitative way of treating human beings.[11]

The view of many Protestant theologians is different. In this line of Christian thinking the sacrosanct nature of very early human embryos is not usually emphasized, and therapeutic cloning, with all its potential benefits to human welfare, is seen as less problematic than reproductive cloning.[12]

I will leave the concept of dignity with the note that human dignity is probably a value held dear by us all. It is a common name given to whatever we value in human life. It is a name for "that something" many of us have a problem putting our finger on. It is not the same for all and, therefore, it is not a very helpful tool in drawing lines between the acceptable and the unacceptable.

4. Is Uniqueness Threatened by Human Cloning?

It has been suggested that humans possess something called "a right to uniqueness," and that this profound right could be violated by cloning.[13] The suggestion is problematic in two obvious respects. The existence of identical twins, and the fact that most cultures do not see a moral problem in their inherited similarity, seems to suggest that even if such a right existed, it would not be absolute, or even very highly valued. Furthermore a clone would in most cases be less of an exact genetic copy of its "sibling" than an identical twin, because the mitochondrial DNA of clones comes from the egg used, not from the nucleus transferred, and this makes the clones, even genetically speaking, unique (unless, of course, the egg and the nucleus are from the same person). Besides, a clone would also be unique, because it would be brought up in a different environment; it would be subject to non-repeatable experiences in changing surroundings; and it would thus develop into an individual of its own.[14]

Despite these problems, attempts have been made to argue that intentionally creating a genetic copy of a human being would violate the right to uniqueness, although the existence of identical twins does not. Most people holding this view seem to believe that the uniqueness of identical twins is based on their "natural" or "God-given" origins. For instance, Donald Bruce states that "[E]ven identical twins are unique [but clones are not]."[15] This apparently follows from the fact that God gives uniqueness to people of his own making, but would deny it to man-made clones. This theological assumption sounds almost too tempting to let go unchallenged, but I will not pursue it further here. Leon Kass, in his turn, argues that there is a moral difference between "natural accidents" and "deliberate human design and manipulation."[16] A similar ethos can also be found in the report of the German Enquete Commission on gene technology.[17]

Even leaving theological elements aside, this argument is not without its difficulties. I cannot but think that the inner logic of the argument must be something like the following. Uniqueness is valuable to people, just like health is valuable to people. Not all people are healthy, but they are nevertheless as worthy as human beings as those who are. There is, however, something wrong about ill-health and, therefore, intentionally making others experience ill-health is wrong. Analogically, although identical twins are as worthy as other people, there is, however, something wrong in not having a unique genetic constitution, and, therefore, intentionally creating identical genotypes is wrong. I dare say that identical twins, and most other people, would disagree with the assumptions underlying this line of thinking. However, the argument from uniqueness only works (at least in a secular setting) if we think that there is something wrong in not having a unique genotype, that is, if we think that there is something wrong in being a twin. But even if we held this rather discriminatory view, it would not follow that clones would be less valuable as persons. It is only if we thought that there is something less valuable about twins *per se* that we could assign a lesser value to clones, too. Since this is not the case, we should conclude that, in the light of this argument, a person born with the help of cloning processes would be as important an individual as those born through the more conventional methods of reproduction.[18]

5. Is Cloning Treating People as a Mere Means?

With the shortcomings of the arguments from uniqueness, many arguments against human reproductive cloning employ the Kantian idea that we should never treat people as a mere means.[19] This has also been expressed in the language of instrumentalization. Those who use this line of argument claim that by intentionally creating a copy of an existing individual, we are treating the produced copy as a mere means, and are not then treating it also as an end in itself, as we should according to the Kantian doctrine.[20] That is, Kant states:

> Humanity itself is a dignity, for man can be used by no one (neither by others nor even by himself) merely as a means, but must always be used at the same time as an end.[21]

It is debatable, however, whether cloning—if used mainly for reproductive purposes—violates the humanity principle any more than any other intentional act of reproduction. I, for one, have never heard of anyone who would have reproduced only for the sake of the forthcoming baby. (There are also some metaphysical problems related to the fact that at the time of the deliberation, nothing of the future child exists.) And, as long as we do not wish to condemn parents for wanting to have children, it would be hypocritical to condemn those who wish to use cloning as an infertility treatment.

If, however, people use reproductive cloning to "bring back a lost loved one" or to recreate any other person they for some reason think of as worth recreating, the accusation of going against the humanity principle might stick. If we do not believe in simple genetic determinism and think that a person's uniqueness is a sum of different factors, many of which are nongenetic, the idea that we could bring back someone is simply wrong—wrong in the sense that it cannot be done. If it were, however, attempted, and the person created by cloning treated, not as a person of her own, but as (a recreation of) someone else, that would indeed count as treating the clone as a mere means. In these circumstances cloning would violate the humanity principle. It does not, however, follow that human reproductive cloning *per se* would be a violation of the principle.[22]

The "treating people as a mere means" argument works unconditionally against therapeutic cloning *if* we believe that early embryos are "human" in the sense intended in the principle.[23] To use early embryos solely for the benefit of others would be to treat them as a mere means. On the other hand, if we do not see early embryos as "human," the condemnation of therapeutic cloning on the basis of treating the embryos as a mere means does not apply (in the sense intended by the "humanity principle").

6. Dangers and Other Costs

There are a number of other practical arguments presented against human reproductive cloning. First of all, the method is not safe. It took 277 attempts to fuse a nucleus with an egg to make Dolly, the cloned sheep. In the subsequent attempts to clone animals it has become clear that at least the "large offspring syndrome," respiratory distress, circulatory problems, kidney and brain malformation, and immune dysfunction are problems typically experienced by cloned mammals. It is to be expected that human clones would display similar lethal or potentially lethal conditions.[24] It goes without saying that for those who hold any human "material" to be sacred, just the loss of eggs and early embryos would be an unacceptable price to pay.

Even if a more liberal stand is taken on the moral status of the early embryos—even if it is held that they have very little or no moral value—the price of cloning in terms of human suffering seems intolerably high. Research leading to human cloning and every attempt to clone a human would require quite a number of donated eggs. This would necessitate a lot of women agreeing to undergo hormone treatments and egg harvesting—neither of which is very pleasant, nor without risks. Informed consent would, perhaps, in the light of current medical ethics and ethics of research, make this acceptable, even if questions can be asked about the justification for such research. Also, both the research and actual attempts to bring cloned human fetuses to term would require a lot of women volunteers to carry the fetuses. Again, the needed hormonal treatments, pregnancy, and childbirth are not without risks. But if the women, of their own free will, wish to participate, that is acceptable within the liberal framework. The women involved are autonomous agents who can give their consent to the procedures. It can be argued, though, that if the need for volunteers grows significantly, the risk of exploitation is also likely to increase. It is, however, the clones themselves who do not have any say in the matter, until it is too late.

There are a number of difficulties in dealing with the rights of those who do not yet exist, and perhaps never will, and the duties we have towards them.[25] What can be said is that attempts to clone human beings will, to the best of our knowledge, result in a large number of births of suffering individuals.[26] It is yet to be established what the great benefits justifying human reproductive cloning in the face of this outcome would be. I will deal with its potential benefits in the next section.

In terms of research ethics, it might be that research into human cloning cannot (ever) be justified, even if there is nothing absolutely wrong with human cloning as such. According to the leading scientists the technique cannot be adequately tested on other mammals, because species seem to react differently to the practice. On the other hand, it seems likely that, as with other mammals, many human clones could have lethal defects that become visible only after their birth.[27] No ethics committee would allow controlled trials on cloning up to the time after birth. It is only very early embryos on which experiments are allowed. It might be that human cloning remains a mere possibility, because research into it cannot be permitted. And we can only hope that, with the expected risks, nobody will attempt to clone humans without prior research.

In addition to the direct human suffering, research into human reproductive cloning can arguably cause suffering indirectly. The trials are, it is to be presumed, very costly. With the number of eggs, wombs, drugs, skilled personnel, and high-tech equipment needed, the money could perhaps be better spent elsewhere.[28]

7. Cloning as Rights Satisfaction, and Other Expected Benefits of Human Reproductive Cloning

In what follows, I will have to assume, against current knowledge and predictions, that the technique of cloning can be perfected without serious violations of accepted codes of research ethics. Otherwise, thorny issues concerning our right to benefit from past evil deeds would arise.[29]

Among the most favorably envisaged future uses of human reproductive cloning is that of helping infertile couples to have a child of "their" genetic heritage. The argument for this is backed up with the idea of what some call the right to reproduce, or reproductive freedom. The right to start a family is, after all, one of the internationally acclaimed Human Rights.[30] It is argued that since everyone has the right to reproduce, research into reproductive cloning should be funded publicly to help even more people who are currently suffering from infertility.

The alleged right to reproduce is, however, a complicated notion, and has been interpreted in numerous ways around the world. To start with, it is not clear who possesses such a right.[31] In many countries the reading is that, in the end, the woman should have a stronger say in the matter. Many countries allow women to decide on abortions on their own, so, it can be argued, depriving men of even the bare liberty to reproduce without interference from others.[32] And as for individuals with severe learning difficulties, and people who have been institutionalized, while their routine sterilization is no longer condoned in the West, their reproductive freedom is still in many respects severely limited.

The paragon right holders here are fertile women and fertile men who engage in traditional heterosexual penetrative sex with each other. Their right to reproduce is a solid liberty right with which nobody should normally interfere. (The most notable exceptions include women's abortion rights, the right to use contraceptives, and prohibitions concerning incest, rape, and deception.) If there are fertility problems, or difficulties in finding a suitable partner, the right to reproduce is reduced into a privilege. It is then up to the proper authorities to decide who is worthy of exercising the right to reproduce. Sometimes the privilege is granted more readily to the wealthy, as in countries with public health care systems there is a difference between the services that are provided, paid for, or compensated by the state, on the one hand and the services that have to be purchased privately on the other. Also, the wealthy are often viewed as more likely to be able to provide a good home for their child, and consequently are desirable candidates for the public services too. It seems clear that the modern world has interpreted the "right to reproduce" either as a liberty right or as a privilege, and that there is no general positive right for everyone to have children. (By a "positive right to x," I mean that someone has a duty to see to it that x comes about, or is realized.[33]) From this it follows, at least, that there is no public duty to fund research into human cloning.

It is, however, plausible to argue that because the right to reproduce is, nonetheless, a liberty, nobody should interfere with privately funded attempts to clone humans. And it may be unfair to pick on cloning, when the alternative does not fare much better in comparison. The uncontrolled exercise of the right to reproduce by those who have the "natural" means at their disposal has caused, and continues to cause, unbearable suffering. Children are born in terrible conditions, they are neglected, abused, subjected to dangerous substances even before birth, and in many cases simply not cared for. The right to reproduce as a liberty has, however, been thought to be so important to what it means to be human that all the suffering it causes is accepted as a price worth paying.

Those who wish to hold on to the right to reproduce, but who wish to ban cloning, have pointed out that cloning is not reproduction in the sense intended by the right, because it is asexual.[34] There are two main objections that can be made to this claim. The first is to ask, who or what authority has defined the conceptually acceptable modes of reproduction? The other is to argue that even if to have a child through cloning would not fall under the "right to reproduce," the unrestricted freedom of individuals to do what they choose, unless they harm others, is usually accepted in liberal societies. Under this "right to autonomy" principle, people could use cloning for reproductive purposes—if nobody is harmed in the process. The terms of the "if" clause are, in the light of what we now know about cloning, difficult to meet.

Another suggested positive outcome of human reproductive cloning is the possibility of avoiding certain mitochondrial diseases. The mitochondria we inherit comes only from the mother, and if the mother has a mitochondrial disease, it will be passed on to her children. If the process of nuclear transfer could be mastered, a couple could have their own (mitochondrial-disease-free) genetic offspring by using an egg from a donor. This would involve fertilizing the woman's egg with the man's sperm, then transferring the nucleus into an egg with healthy mitochondria, and finally implanting this egg in the woman's uterus.[35] This practice would, I assume, meet with far less resistance than other types of human reproductive cloning. It would not involve making a copy of another human being, and the social parents of the child would be almost entirely its genetic parents as well. It should be noted, though, that mitochondrial diseases are relatively rare, and it could take a long time before nuclear transfer can be done to the precision needed for this to work. Meanwhile, however, research into human cloning is likely to produce a lot of suffering, and it is by no means evident that a possible future method of avoiding mitochondrial diseases would justify all this.

8. Cast Shadows? Denied Ignorance? Closed Future?

So far I have concentrated on the general wrongs associated with cloning, and have only dealt with the well-being of the clones in terms of the potential health effects of the procedure. It is now time to consider what it would be like to be a clone. Would there be something wrong with that?

It has been argued that even if clones were full human persons, their lives might still be deprived of certain important aspects of human life, which would make intentional attempts to clone humans wrong. It has been suggested that a clone would live its life in the shadow of the human from whom it was cloned,[36] and that the clone would be denied the right to ignorance.[37] Some have claimed that Joel Feinberg's argument from "the child's right to an open future" would also carry the same message.[38] Feinberg's argument is not, however, as such, applicable to genetic manipulation or cloning, because it is focused on the child's open future in relation to its "natural" (genetically fixed) potential, and does not therefore address the futures of individuals who may, on genetic grounds, never exist.[39]

The idea of the "life in the shadow" and "right to ignorance" arguments is that although it is relatively clear that our identity and personhood are not straightforwardly determined by our genes, it is possible that certain expectations are projected onto "cloned lives" by the individuals living those lives, or by other people. The life in the shadow argument emphasizes the expected fact that others would look at clones comparing them to the originals, and the ignorance argument draws mostly on the existential experiences of the clones themselves as people who have been (or who believe they have been) foretold their destiny.[40]

A life in the shadow of another human being would, arguably, "diminish the clone's possibility of living a life that is in a full sense of that word his or her life."[41] Insofar as people are, even partly, perceived as living other people's (more original) lives, this is bad for them as persons of their own. This argument shows that as long as people have a tendency to see clones as mere shadows of their originals, there is something wrong with cloning. It is another question, however, whether this observed tendency can prove that cloning should be prohibited. It is debatable whether the shadow of the original on a clone is any worse than the shadow cast by many ("ordinary") parents on their children.

The idea that cloning is wrong because it produces human beings who know too much (or believe that they know too much) about themselves, relies on the existential idea that life is about discovering oneself.[42] The wrongness of cloning, according to those who hold this view, lies in the fact that clones are not given the chance (when they know of the original) fully to discover themselves, as some of the finding out has already been done by the original. This argument, too, draws on the assumed fact that people would lean towards genetic determinism in their view of themselves, or others, as clones. Leaving the existential issues on one side, a case against cloning could be attempted by appeals to the argument that people have a right to ignorance regarding their own genetic makeup.[43]

If we assume that there is such a right as that to genetic ignorance, it does seem that cloning is wrong because it violates this right. If the cloned persons are in contact with the originals, and the originals are significantly older than the clones, then the clones would have a lesser degree of ignorance about their genetic makeups than other people do. Then, again, the question is, what type of a right is the right to genetic ignorance?[44] Given the fact that people cannot be adequately protected against genetic information in any case—they only need to look in the mirror or meet their blood relatives to know something about their genetic makeup—it would seem that the right to genetic ignorance can only be a negative claim right. By a negative claim right I mean that the right-holder has no duty to know about her own genetic makeup, and that others have a duty not to inform her (against her own wishes).[45] A right like this does not, however, obligate others actively to protect her from the information. I would be tempted to think that cloning does not violate the right to genetic ignorance as a negative claim right, although the issue is debatable.

9. Odds and Ends

In addition to the main arguments against cloning that I have studied here, there are numerous other issues that are often brought up in discussions of the topic. For instance, some are worried about the impoverishment of the human gene pool should cloning become a regular method of reproduction. Others bring up the difficulties all this causes to family and social life; where a mother can also be a sister and one's grandparents can also be one's genetic parents. The clones depicted in sci-fi literature have also left their mark on people's views on cloning. A persistent image seems to be one involving armies of less-than-human clones marching in step. This seems to keep alive the notion of clones as beings that have been created to serve an evil purpose or to do a dubious or inhumane job.

It is unlikely that cloning will ever become the main method of reproduction, and even if it did, the human gene pool would not be threatened for a long time. As for the changes in family life, the one-size-fits-all family model with two parents of opposite sexes and their own genetic offspring has for some time now been a thing of the past. There are no particular reasons to expect that people could not assimilate children from yet another source into their lives. As for the fear of eugenics, I would not think that a new technology that, in theory, makes possible certain types of eugenics, would force societies to adopt eugenic policies. We already have the technology to screen fetuses, test prospective parents, sterilize people, and abort unwanted pregnancies. We have the means to large-scale eugenics, but we do not choose to use them. I would think it plausible to argue that it is the socio-political atmosphere that determines how these methods, and in the future possibly cloning, are used, and not the technology that determines the socio-political views.

However, the fact that people are horrified by cloning should not be dismissed too lightly. The idea of human cloning causes significant fear and distress in many people, and those anxieties, too, should be addressed as one of the "costs" of cloning—even if the fears could be shown to be ungrounded, and despite the fact that "yuk" reactions are not usually recognized as moral arguments.[46] This is especially so when there seems to be precious little reason for attempting human reproductive cloning in the first place.

10. Surprisingly Little Wrong, But Still . . . . Conclusion

As far as we know, we can expect very marginal benefits from human reproductive cloning. It could be used as an alternative fertility treatment, and the method of nuclear transfer could be used to avoid some mitochondrial diseases, but with no generally acknowledged positive right to reproduce and with the rarity of mitochondrial diseases, it is far from clear that we should use cloning to tackle these issues. The arguments presented against human reproductive cloning do not, at least philosophically speaking, unequivocally justify an absolute condemnation of human re-productive cloning, but the cumulative effect of the contingent wrongs related to the practice should make us wary, to say the least.

Research leading to human reproductive cloning would not only require trials on very early embryos, but it would require carrying some fetuses to term as well. With the expected risks, research proposals on cloning would not gain ethical approval. Without proper research, to attempt human reproductive cloning, again with the associated risks, would be wrong. It does seem that unless the outstanding safety issues on research into human cloning can be addressed, we cannot conduct the necessary research, and, consequently, cannot justifiably attempt human reproductive cloning.

Human reproductive cloning is a high-risk, expensive enterprise with, even in the best-case scenario, only minor benefits. It is not an absolute wrong, and should not be condemned as such. However, because, as it now seems, the safety issues cannot be resolved, and research into human cloning would cause suffering and place the study subjects under unacceptable risk, it should not, as things now stand, be attempted. And even if the safety issues could, sometime in the future, be properly addressed, it would be wrong to invest public money into research with so few benefits to human welfare (provided that the money could be used for more worthy causes elsewhere).

NOTES

1. Ian Wilmut, A. A. Schnieke, J. McWhir, A. J. Kind, and K. H. S. Campbell., "Viable Offspring Derived from Fetal and Adult Mammalian Cells," *Nature*, 385 (1997), pp. 810–813.

2. See, e.g., UNESCO *Universal Declaration on the Human Genome and Human Rights*, UNESCO, 3 Dec 1997; The European Parliament, *Resolution on Cloning*, 13 Mar 1997; National Bioethics Advisory Commission, *1996-1997 Annual Report*, Maryland, USA, March 1998, Appendix B.

3. Søren Holm, "A Life in the Shadow: One Reason Why We Should Not Clone Humans," *Cambridge Quarterly of Healthcare Ethics*, 7:2 (Spring 1998), pp. 160–162.

4. See e.g. Pontificia Acedemia Pro Vita, *Reflections on Cloning* (Vatican: Libreria Editrice Vaticana, 1997).

5. Rebecca Kolberg., "Human Embryo Cloning Reported," *Science* 262:5134 (29 October 1993), pp. 652–653.

6. Alan Colman, "Why Human Cloning Should Not Be Attempted," *The Genetic Revolution and Human Rights*, ed. Justine Burley (Oxford: Oxford University Press, 1999), p. 15.

7. See e.g. UNESCO, *Universal Declaration on Human Genome and Human Rights*; Council of Europe, *Additional Protocol to the Convention for the Protection of Human Rights and Dignity of the Human Being with Regard to the Application of Biology and Medicine, on the Prohibition of Cloning Human Beings (with additional Explanatory Report)*. European treaties ETS No. 168 DIR/JUR (98)7; cf. United Nations, general Assembly 11 November 2002, *International Convention Against the Reproductive Cloning of Human Beings*, Report of the Sixth Committee, Draft Resolution A/C.6/57/L.3/Rev.1 and Corr.1.

8. See e.g. John Harris, "Clones, Genes, and Human Rights," *The Genetic Revolution and Human Rights*, ed. Burley, pp. 66–67; cf. Matti Häyry, "Another Look at Dignity," *Cambridge Quarterly of Healthcare Ethics*, 13:1 (2004), pp. 7–14.

9. David de Pomerai, "Dolly Mixtures: Retrospects and Prospects for Animal and Human Cloning," *Journal of Genetics and Ethics*, 4:2 (1998), p. 46.

10. Donald Bruce, "Cloning—A Step Too Far," *Journal of Genetics and Ethics*, 4:2 (1998), p. 37.

11. Pontificia Academia Pro Vita, 1997, 15 & 14.

12. Bruce, "Cloning—A Step Too Far"; *Ethical Issues in Human Stem Cell Research, Volume III: Religious Approaches* (Rockville, MD: National Bioethics Advisory Commission, June 2000).

13. See e.g. UNESCO, *Universal Declaration on the Human Genome and Human Rights*, 1997.

14. Holm, "A Life in the Shadow," p. 160; Dan W. Brock, "Cloning Human Beings: An Assessment of the Ethical Issues Pro and Con," *Clones and Clones: Facts and Fantasies About Human Cloning*, ed. Martha Nussbaum and Cass R. Sunstein (New York: W. W. Norton, 1998), pp. 103–104.

15. Bruce, "Cloning—A Step Too Far," p. 37.

16. Leon R. Kass, *Life, Liberty, and the Defence of Dignity* (San Francisco, CA: Encounter Books, 2002), p. 154.

17. Anon., "A Report from Germany—an Extract from *Prospects and Risks of Gene Technology: The Report of the Enquete Commission to the Bundestag of the Federal Republic of Germany*," *Bioethics* 2 (1988), pp. 256–263. Cf. Ruth Chadwick, "Cloning," *Philosophy* 57 (1982), pp. 201–209.

18. See e.g. Helga Kuhse and Peter Singer, "The Moral Status of the Embryo," *Unsanctifying Human Life: Essays on Ethics*, ed. Helga Kuhse (Oxford: Blackwell, 2002), p. 186.

19. See e.g. Immanuel Kant, *The Metaphysics of Morals*, reprinted in Immanuel Kant, *Practical Philosophy*, ed. Mary J. Gregor (Cambridge: Cambridge University Press, 1996), p. 6:462, § 38. Also, in the same collection, Immanuel Kant, *The Metaphysical Principles of Virtue*, §§ 434–435.

20. See e.g. Hilary Putnam, "Cloning People," *The Genetic Revolution and Human Rights*, ed. Burley, p. 9; John Harris, "'Goodbye Dolly?' The Ethics of Human Cloning," *Journal of Medical Ethics*, 23:6 (1997), p. 355; Harris, "Clones, Genes, and Human Rights," pp. 67–78.

21. Kant, *The Metaphysics of Morals*, p. 6:462.

22. John Harris, "Is Cloning an Attack on Human Dignity?," *Nature*, 387:6635 (19 June 1997), p. 754; K. Labib, "Don't Leave Dignity Out of the Cloning Debate," *Nature*, 388:6637 (3 July 1997), p. 15; A. Kahn, "Cloning, Dignity, and Ethical Revisionism," *Nature*, 388:6640 (24 July 1997), pp. 320; D. Shapiro, "Cloning, Dignity, and Ethical reasoning," *Nature*, 388:6642 (7 August 1997), p. 511; John Harris, "Cloning and Bioethical Thinking," *Nature*, 389:6640 (2 October 1997), p. 433.

23. Cf., however, Immanuel Kant, *The Metaphysical Principles of Virtue*, §§ 434–435, and *Groundwork of the Metaphysics of Morals*, pp. 439–440, in the same collection.

24. Ian Wilmut, "Dolly: The Age of Biological Control," *The Genetic Revolution and Human Rights*, ed. Burley, p. 20; R. Jaenisch and Ian Wilmut, "Don't Clone Humans," *Science*, 291:5513 (30 March 2001), p. 2552.

25. Cf., however, Derek Parfit, *Reasons and Persons* (Oxford: Oxford University Press, 1984); Justine Burley and John Harris, "Human Cloning and Child Welfare," *Journal of Medical Ethics*, 25:2 (April 1999), pp. 109–110; D. McCarthy, "Persons and their Copies," *Journal of Medical Ethics*, 25:2 (April 1999), pp. 99–100.

26. See e.g. Jaenisch and Wilmut, "Don't Clone Humans."

27. *Ibid.*

28. See Immaculada de Melo-Martín, "On Cloning Human Beings," *Bioethics*, 16:3 (2002), pp. 254–265.

29. See e.g. Tuija Takala and Matti Häyry, "Benefiting from Past Wrongdoing, Human Embryonic Stem Cell Lines, and the Fragility of the German Legal Position," *Ethics of Stem Cells*, ed. John Harris (Oxford: Oxford University Press, forthcoming).

30. United Nations, *Universal Declaration of Human Rights*. Adopted by the General Assembly on 10 December 1948.

31. See e.g. Kass, *Life, Liberty, and the Defence of Dignity*, p. 163; Ruth Deech, "Cloning and Public Policy," *The Genetic Revolution and Human Rights*, ed. Burley, pp. 95–100.

32. See e.g. Joel Feinberg, *Social Philosophy* (Englewood Cliffs, N.J.: Prentice Hall, 1973), pp. 55–67.

33. *Ibid.*

34. See e.g. Kass, *Life, Liberty, and the Defence of Dignity*; Deech, "Cloning and Public Policy."

35. Wilmut, "Dolly: The Age of Biological Control," pp. 23–24.

36. Holm, "A Life in the Shadow."

37. Hans Jonas, "Biological Engineering—A Preview," *Philosophical Essays: From Ancient Creed to Technological Man* (Englewood Cliffs, N.J.: Prentice-Hall, 1974) 141–167.

38. E.g., Brock, "Cloning Human Beings: An Assessment of the Ethical Issues Pro and Con"; also de Melo-Martín, "On Cloning Human Beings," p. 250; Joel Feinberg, "The Child's Right to an Open Future," in his *Freedom and Fulfillment: Philosophical Essays* (Princeton: Princeton University Press, 1992), pp. 76–97.

39. See e.g. Tuija Takala, "The Child's Right to an Open Future and Modern Genetics," *Ethical Issues in the New Genetics: Are Genes Us?*, ed. Brenda Almond and Michael Parker (Aldershot: Ashgate, 2003), pp. 39–46.

40. Holm, "A Life in the Shadow"; Jonas, "Biological Engineering."

41. Holm "A Life in the Shadow," p. 162.

42. Jonas, "Biological Engineering," pp. 159–163.

43. See e.g. Tuija Takala, "The Right to Ignorance Confirmed," *Bioethics*, 13:3–4 (July 1999), pp. 288–293; Matti Häyry and Tuija Takala, "Genetic Ignorance, Moral Obligations, and Social Duties," *Journal of Medicine and Philosophy*, 25:1 (February 2000), pp. 107–113; Matti Häyry, and Tuija Takala, "Genetic Information, Rights and Autonomy," *Theoretical Medicine and Bioethics*, 22:5 (September 2001), pp. 403–414; Tuija Takala, "Genetic Ignorance and Reasonable Paternalism," *Theoretical Medicine and Bioethics*, 22:5 (September 2001), pp. 485–491.

44. Cf. Feinberg, *Social Philosophy*; Häyry and Takala, "Genetic Information, Rights, and Autonomy."

45. Häyry and Takala, "Genetic Information, Rights, and Autonomy."

46. See e.g. Jonathan Glover, "Eugenics and Human Rights," *The Genetic Revolution and Human Rights*, ed. Burley, pp. 101–104; cf. Kass, *Life, Liberty, and the Defence of Dignity*, p. 150.

Six

THE PROBLEM OF INTANGIBLES

Louise Irving

1. Introduction

Most approaches to contemporary problems, if they are to be taken seriously, are justified by some manner of measurement. Bioethics is particularly important, as the development of policy and regulation in this area has considerable consequences. Advances in scientific and genetic technology bring with them the problem of insufficient knowledge of consequences and a public already alarmed about the fallibility of science and cynical about assurances. The potential good of something like stem cell research and genetic screening tends to fall under the same scientific umbrella as fears about the genetic modification of crops and cloning in raising public alarm. It is difficult to know whether public outcry about some of these advances indicates a proper area for concern, or is merely a reflection of knee-jerk reactions to the new. Much of this public outcry is labeled as the "yuk" factor—"we do not like it, but we are not sure why." There is a struggle to express what the problem may be, with vague talk of procedures being "against nature," and concern about the erosion of respect for human dignity and uniqueness. There does seem to be an intuitive understanding that there are things important to personhood and human flourishing like dignity and equal respect for persons. But these are often difficult to articulate and therefore to quantify, so consideration of them is generally not an issue.

In order for bioethics to be considered effective as a discipline, it needs to be comprehensive in its approach to bioethical problems. Part of this approach would perhaps require analysis of existing relevant empirical research and theoretical concepts which would be considered alongside the usual ethical frameworks and principles. To consider how a more holistic approach to problems in bioethics might look, it is helpful to start with a case in which widely accepted moral principles alone lead to conclusions that may appear to be morally counter-intuitive. I illustrate with a case study, but the argument is broadly applicable to bioethical problems in general. The case study relates to a commercial trade in kidneys, and the argument in favor of allowing such a trade is said to be made through logic and analysis rather than any particular rights-based or libertarian positions. This type of philosophical argument may look as if it stands on its own, easily dismissing the "yuk" factor as an unsubstantiated reaction. But, perhaps the "yuk" factor does indicate something substantive, and it may be possible to assess this by factoring in "the world as it is," instead of merely using abstract moral principles ("the world as it should be") as a reference point.

2. The Case for Commerce

In 1989, two British surgeons were exposed in a scandal involving the buying of kidneys from Turkish nationals to treat private patients in the United Kingdom. This caused a huge public outcry, and legislation—in the form of the Human Organ Transplant Act (1989)—was swiftly introduced to ban the practice. However, there has since been a call by The International Forum for Transplant Ethics for this ban to be reviewed. The Forum asks us to consider the following argument.[1]

There is very little in existing law to support prohibition, and indeed the reaction of widespread repugnance was itself taken as justification for the ban. The law already permits persons to make extreme choices regarding what they do with their bodies. For example, a person can refuse medical treatment even if death is a certain outcome. The legislation on abortion and non-therapeutic sterilization and the legality of (often extreme) cosmetic surgery procedures all imply that our bodies are, in a sense, our property to decide what to do with.

The concern about a commercial trade in kidneys was that it could involve exploitation of the poor, and altruistic donation was used as the legal demarcation line to prevent this from happening. This distinction is based upon the doctrine of consent, which must be informed and voluntary for surgical intervention to be valid. It was assumed that financial inducement prevents uncoerced consent. But the Forum argues, logically and correctly, that this is an unsafe distinction. There is nothing to suggest that a person cannot make an informed choice to sell a kidney for an altruistic reason, and this was indeed the case for one of the Turkish nationals in the original scandal. He was raising money to pay for an operation for his daughter. Also, altruistic donations may be coercive through the pressure of expectation, guilt, or obligation, and these pressures can be even greater than any perceived financial inducement. The risk to the donor is minimal, an immediate post-op risk of 0.05% and a 0.07% chance of something happening to the remaining kidney.[2] This is deemed perfectly acceptable for altruistic donors, so arguing against kidney sales on the grounds of risk is ineffective. Finally, even if we think kidney selling is wrong, it does not follow that prohibition is warranted. *The Warnock Committee Report into Surrogacy* unanimously disapproved of the practice.[3] Despite this, it held that prohibition of private arrangements, involving the payment of pretty flexible expenses, was not warranted, on the grounds of the privacy of individuals and the difficulty of enforcement.

The philosophical arguments are similarly straightforward. A main concern is the "slippery slope" argument, which holds that a commercial trade in kidneys might lead to the selling of vital organs. This worry is not valid, since legally you cannot consent to be killed or seriously injured.

There is a question about the validity of consent to selling one's kidneys that has two aspects. The first is that economic coercion precludes informed consent. The Forum concludes that it may be reasonable to say that poverty is forcing people to sell, but that by "protecting" these people we take away the only option they have left, thereby making them less autonomous. The second is that those likely to sell a kidney will not be educated enough to understand the risk and implications of their choice. To this it is answered that these concerns should be addressed by a system of information and counseling, and if this is impracticable then the decision should be in the hands of a guardian, as is the situation under law. The International Forum for Transplant Ethics states that "our indignation on behalf of the exploited poor seems to take the curious form of wanting to make them worse off still."

Arguments in defense of the current prohibition are considered to be much less tangible. They relate to possibilities of a moral decline and corruption of sensibilities if body parts are considered saleable. It is argued that this rhetoric cannot hope to outweigh the very real harms of death and destitution. To say that commodification of the self is wrong is just stating a point instead of giving a reason. The Forum states that:

> [A]ttempts to justify the deep feelings of repugnance … are the real driving force of prohibition, and feelings of repugnance among the rich and healthy, no matter how strongly felt, cannot justify removing the only hope of the destitute and dying.[4]

To summarize the Forum's case: there is an overwhelming need to increase the supply of kidneys, and this can be done at a stroke by lifting the ban. There probably would not even be a ban if legislation had not been rushed through on the wave of a scandal, as no one would argue on the face of the evidence that it was warranted. There are great social gains to be made, both of cost to the health service on a micro-level (less long term dialysis), and in the advancement of autonomy and general well being on a macro-level. We may not like it, but that is no reason for stopping it. The lifting of the ban would reflect a commitment to autonomy and the legal rights entailed by self-determination.

3. Logic versus Intuition

So there we have it: impartial logic and reason at work. And the public outcry and inconsistent legislation can be seen as knee-jerk reactions—the "yuk" factor in operation. We may feel repugnance toward the trade, but commitment to liberal autonomy demands a substantive reason to support prohibition, and we do not have one. The Forum argues that those who say logic must not be placed above moral intuition are refusing to attend to moral questions at all, and if none of the arguments can demonstrate that kidney selling is wrong, then supporters of prohibition, because they somehow feel or intuit something wrong with this practice, are "flailing at logic."

"Intuitionism" is a bit of a bad word in philosophy, and rightly so. The Greeks intuitively "knew" there was nothing wrong with slavery. People "knew" women's brains were smaller than men's (some still "know" this), or that some races were inferior to others. Others are confident they "know" absolutely that homosexuality is morally wrong. So Intuitionism is no guide to moral integrity and we must leave it behind and leave the job to logic and reason.

But what if we still think that something is wrong here? Can the whole of the public outcry, bearing in mind that this practice is almost universally banned, be just misguided? That this is a possibility was pointed out to me by John Harris. However, if we think that there is something counter-intuitive in the conclusion that the poor must be free to sell their body parts and that we do them a disservice by not letting them, we seem to have nothing left with which to argue this point, without being subject to accusations of flailing at logic.

But maybe there is a second-order moral question here—the one which asks why reasoning from logic leads to conclusions that many of us clearly feel are morally suspect. If it is so logically obvious and legally compelling then why is there such a tension about this issue? Is our disquiet telling us something important?

Janet Radcliffe-Richards, writing in support of a commercial trade in kidneys, admits that she feels the same repugnance toward the trade, but that reason has forced her to override this concern.[5] The philosopher Raymond Gaita says that philosophers who say they courageously follow reason where it compels them are often indulging in "self-congratulatory cant."[6] While this seems rather harsh directed against the rationale of potential good advanced by those who see a market in organs as a solution, there is a point here that needs to be elaborated. If logic and reason lead to a conclusion that many feel is nevertheless alarming and wrong, must we merely accept the conclusion? Do we not need to examine the premises? The argument from autonomy is based on one of negative liberty, the right to be left alone to live life as you please unless your actions harm another. As no harm can be found in the private transactions of willing buyers and vendors, the conclusion is that prohibition is unwarranted, undesirable, and paternalistic. It is this conception of liberty that makes rationales like free market solutions logically and legally compelling and, as we can see, morally defensible.

4. The Tendency toward Commodification

So, what are the premises and assumptions that give rise to tension between what seems to be logically correct, and a widespread moral intuition that it is morally suspect? Well, there seem to be at least three things going on here that make the inevitable conclusion one of commodification.

We hold a concept of property as private property plus free contract. The right to property is inalienable (a fundamental right for all) but the property itself is considered fully alienable (we must be able to dispose of our property, events such as bankruptcy aside). So market alienability, the right to sell, is inherent in the concept of property itself. Inalienabilities, things that are outside the market, are then conceptually and normatively problematic. The "conceptualist" view of property cannot hold that some things are property but not fully alienable. It can only hold that some things are just not property.[7]

We do think of the body as property. The normative way we have of speaking about the body is further supported by the way we understand what is "ours." The normative discourse used when talking about the body is one of ownership. Expressions like "it is my body" and "you do not own me" are a manner of speaking rather than an expression of bodily ownership. They reflect the negative right to be left alone that is legally enshrined in the requirement of consent to be touched. But this way of speaking in an increasingly market driven society gives rise to concepts of rights of transfer including buying and selling.[8]

It is generally accepted that liberalism in its broadest sense sees liberty as the absence of restrictions. In other words freedom *is* non-interference. From this it is assumed that respect for autonomy requires good government to avoid stating any preferences regarding the choices and lifestyles of its citizens. These choices may be good, bad, or arbitrary, but the important thing is that they are made by the person. This tends toward commodification, because freedom is defined as individual freedom of choice.

Acceptance of these tenets leads to the conclusion that my kidney is my property, and no one can tell me what the good is for me: property is alienable, therefore I must be allowed to sell it if I wish. So we can see how these basic premises all tend toward commodification, aided and driven by the customary rhetoric of economic analysis, by only being able to measure quantifiable harms. This person is dying, this person is poor, and in this way the language of liberal democracy is becoming indistinguishable from the language of the free market.

5. Freedom as Non-Interference

Peter Singer, in his book on Hegel, writes that negative liberty takes the choices of individuals as its starting point and the mechanism of the market allows these to be realized with no questions asked about how these choices are formed. A *laissez faire* system without direction or morals results in absurdities, and for this reason the success of the market needs to be judged not by its ability to meet the necessarily self-interested choices of individuals, but on its ability to satisfy human needs and welfare.[9]

The freedom of non-interference is worthless without the social and ethical conditions required to make it valuable. Not enquiring into the basis of people's choices absolves us of any responsibility toward those who need protection. The liberal response to this is that we cannot impose our own values on others. The reluctance to interfere can be defended by an unwillingness to be paternalistic. However, as Hegel would argue, there is already a value judgment there—a judgment about the value of action based on choice, regardless of how that choice is reached. For Hegel, negative liberty is the freedom to be manipulated by the particular social and economic circumstances of the time. The acceptance of negative liberty as freedom and the choice of the individual as the only relevant starting point necessitates the conclusions of the Forum. However, good and important values are already written into the liberal ideal and it is simply wrong to say there is no way of judging the desirability of people's choices. This is not to compare homosexuality to heterosexuality, prostitutes to poets, or drug taking to abstinence. It is to look at the basis of the choice, especially when we suspect that it is coerced by circumstances, and determine whether it is valuable to the flourishing of the individual.

So, a commitment to liberal neutrality leads to a particular reading of the facts, and the pervasiveness of the discourse makes it difficult to conceive of the conclusions as substantively wrong. However, if we believe the premises may be flawed, then we are not compelled to accept the conclusion. The premises exemplify a discourse that is detrimental, since it enforces wrong conceptions of what it is to be free. The idea that people would choose to alienate certain things, a kidney in this context, assumes that alienation—the freedom to sell anything—is an act or enhancement of freedom. If we follow this logic, then everything is up for grabs. However, if we accept that we are driven toward these conclusions by the logic of a discourse then we are entitled to say in advance, from the best conception of things important to personhood, what should be free from market forces. An acceptance of a positive conception of liberty would mean that inalienabilities required to foster self-development would be seen to enhance rather than constrain freedom.

6. Universal Principles in an Unjust World

The one-size-fits-all argument of universal moral principles does not work when addressing the reality of different social and cultural constraints. Japan has no cadaver program largely because of the unacceptability of brain stem death. India likewise has no cadaver program, and financial and organizational problems make long-term dialysis unsuitable. There are particular reasons for these problems that deserve a separate analysis. However, India's particular problems make it an appropriate framework for a one-dimensional analysis, being a society which, arguably, could most benefit from a commercial trade. The argument against prohibition will therefore seem most persuasive against the backdrop of problems such as those in the third world, as the Forum's talk of starving children and destitution attests. But using the argument from autonomy to support it where no such thing, in the true meaning of the word, exists, is flawed. Two desperately bad choices do not amount to autonomy. Those with different religious or cultural constraints will have a different moral framework to argue from and it is questionable that it is our job, in the West, to morally justify a commercial trade for them.

The argument advanced by the International Forum for Transplant Ethics relies on legal analogies and the philosophical commitments to autonomy and informed consent. It is important to keep in mind that those who wish to keep prohibition in place, for whatever reason, are not single-handedly "removing the only hope of the destitute and dying" as was the Forum's accusation. If this were the case, then defenders of prohibition could not bear the moral weight of that argument. But the claim to moral and legal legitimacy of a commercial trade in kidneys rests on the assumption that the problems are caused by the constraints of altruistic donation, and empirical data tells us this is not necessarily the case. It is the alternative methods of organ procurement that a commercial trade in kidneys needs to be weighed against. The Forum may have reached different conclusions if existing data had been taken into account.

7. A Less Ethically Problematic Option

For both the United States and the United Kingdom, the most promising method would be a system of "required response." All adults would be required to register their willingness or refusal to donate through a public authority or their General Practitioner. The administration of such a policy is not thought to be particularly problematic, and all donors could be registered on a central database. This would legally protect the organ procurement organizations, stop next of kin refusals, and maintain the individual's prerogative to opt in, opt out, or delegate the choice to her next of kin. The expectation is that this system would evolve into one of *de facto* presumed consent through familiarization with, and approval of, organ donation. The policy implementation would coincide with a public education campaign to deal with any concerns. A joint National Kidney Foundation and United States' United Network for Organ Sharing survey found that the majority of people who were not registered donors cited the reason that they had never been asked.

Furthermore, focus on an organ shortfall helps to conceal woefully inadequate funding resulting in a lack of facilities and shortage of trained staff which, according to the Royal College of Surgeons, is as much a problem as is organ shortage.[10] There are ways to increase the shortfall in organs which do not suffer the concerns of a commercial trade. These have not benefited from the political will and co-ordination required to make them effective. The law is committed to the formalisms of the political structure, such as the principle of autonomy, while not being able to say what "the good" is for people because of the commitment to liberal neutrality. So there is a tension between the rhetoric and what might perhaps be thought of as a more holistic type of justice. Really the law should probably accept kidney sales. It would accord with the language and conception of bodily ownership and reflect the primacy of the principles of autonomy and consent. But it does not accept it because that widespread abhorrence, the "yuk" factor, means many things. It represents fears of the market encroaching upon, and determining, every area of our lives—even the inside of our bodies; these are fears because, at heart, we know that those with the *least* autonomy will sell. They are fears because intangibles like dignity, bodily integrity, personhood, and flourishing, which we can conceive of but have problems defining, cannot be measured to the satisfaction of a discourse, so are not counted.

It seems to be of incalculable importance to take into account actual knowledge and information about the social world, and not to rely on abstract moral principles to do all the work. We cannot let "reason," whose terms are dictated by a particular framework of discourse that may be impoverished to begin with, decide, or we get impoverished conclusions. Moral philosophy is surely able to propose that that there *is* a conception of the good that demands certain inalienabilities. Acceptance of the empty formalisms of a liberal market economy constrains our ability to think outside market terms. This erodes social responsibility and we further abuse the unfortunate, under the guise of help, by insisting that they must be entitled to make money any way they can.

8. Conclusion

To summarize: we can see how logic and analysis, because located in a particular framework of discourse, necessitate conclusions that can be morally counter-intuitive. The concern about a commercial trade in kidneys is real. But it is difficult to counter the logical argument because the concerns are intangible, and consequently unquantifiable. Cost-benefit analysis is at serious risk of error because it cannot take into account the subjective well being of persons and changes in the way we perceive the world. Other perspectives in moral and political philosophy, such as the Hegelian one, can argue that the premises are flawed, but major changes in the political set-up are not going to be forthcoming. However, issues that arouse such widespread public concern can be examined, and if they are found to be indicative of something substantive, less ethically problematic conclusions can be reached. This requires something more than armchair philosophy—it requires an engagement with social reality.

Even if the argument in favor of a commercial trade in kidneys is rational and logical, this does not necessarily make it ethical. Better and much less morally contentious options are available but are not being recommended. The framework used by the International Forum for Transplant Ethics was far too simple and one-dimensional to fit the social world. Such widespread unease and distaste about a concern in applied ethics should be given more weight—why swim against the tide? Bob Brecher writes that, "the horror of kidney selling is so strong because it symbolizes so absolutely all the wrongs we feel free to ignore because of our familiarity with them."[11]

This is important. It may be, and I believe that it is, that market inalienabilities are needed to engender altruism and keep intact concepts of personhood such as dignity and bodily integrity. If we agree these intangibles are probably important, then ignoring them will not make for a better applied ethics, or a better social reality.

Acknowledgement

The research for this paper has been supported by the Empirical Methods in Bioethics (EMPIRE) project, funded by the European Commission, D-G Research. I thank the commission for its support.

NOTES

1. Janet Radcliffe-Richards, A. S. Daar, R. D. Guttmann, R. Hoffenberg, I. Kennedy, M. Lock, R. A. Sells, and N. Tilney for the International Forum for Transplant Ethics, "The Case for Allowing Kidney Sales," *The Lancet*, 351:9120 (27 June 1998), pp. 1950–1952.

2. Gerald Dworkin, "The Law Relating to Organ Transplantation in England," *Medical Law*, ed. Ian Kennedy and Andrew Grubb (London: Butterworths, 3rd ed., 2000), p. 1084.

3. Baroness Warnock "A Question of Life," *Medical Law*, ed. Kennedy and Grubb, p. 825.

4. Radcliffe-Richards et al, "The Case for Allowing Kidney Sales."

5. Janet Radcliffe-Richards, "Nephrarious Goings on: Kidney Sales and Moral Arguments," *Journal of Medicine and Philosophy*, 21:4 (August 1996), pp. 375-416.

6. Raymond Gaita, *Good and Evil: An Absolute Conception* (Basingstoke: Macmillan, 1991), p. 317.

7. Margaret Jane Radin, "Market Inalienability," *Harvard Law Review*, 100:8 (1987), pp. 1849-1937.

8. Jim Harris "Who Owns My Body," *Oxford Journal of Legal Studies*, 16:1 (Spring 1996), pp. 55–84.

9. Peter Singer, *Hegel* (Oxford: Oxford University Press, 1983), p. 27.

10. Royal College of Surgeons of England, *Report of the Working Party to Review Organ Transplantation* (London: Royal College of Surgeons of England, 1999).

11. Bob Brecher, "The Kidney Trade: Or, the Customer is Always Wrong," *Journal of Medical Ethics*, 16:3 (September 1990), pp. 120–123.

Seven

MIND THE GAP: THE USE OF EMPIRICAL EVIDENCE IN BIOETHICS

Eve Garrard and Stephen Wilkinson

1. Introduction

Is empirical information a significant part of bioethics? On the face of it, the answer to this is so obviously "yes" that there does not seem to be any room for debate. How could any branch of applied ethics be entirely *a priori*? No matter what background ethical theory is endorsed, it seems that the way the world is, empirically speaking, must be relevant to the first-order deliverances of the theory. But this question can be seen as just one example in a long tradition of querying the relation between the world of experience and the world of moral-philosophical reasoning. As far back as classical Greece, Plato was suggesting that the empirical world, including what most people believe about it, had little to offer the philosopher,[1] whereas Aristotle saw respectable opinion about moral matters as an indispensable element in moral theorizing.[2] More recently, a common source of doubt about the relevance of the empirical to the moral has been located in the gap which purportedly exists between facts and values; a gap which defeats, so it is said, any attempt to derive ethical conclusions from empirical premises. And if we cannot derive ethical conclusions from them, the role of empirical data in bioethics appears suspect.

In this chapter, we argue that even if there is a fact-value gap, it does not rule out the relevance of empirical information to ethical debates, and that there are quite strong arguments for thinking that the gap is less wide than it is normally claimed to be, in which case there is little to preclude a close relationship between the empirical data and bioethics. However, it does not follow from this general thought that all kinds of empirical data are able to enter equally into ethical debate. We distinguish between data that are relevant to ethics, and data that are actually part of ethics, and argue that which of these roles is being played by any given piece of empirical information will be a highly context-sensitive matter. We also argue that it is theory-sensitive, because data that are merely *relevant* on an objectivist account of ethics could be construed as *part* of ethics on a relativist account.

Later on, we discuss four particular sources of empirical data: natural science; social science research into the outcomes of our policies and actions; social science research into the behavior and attitudes of ethicists; and social science research into public attitudes. Since, as we argue, relativism is an implausible moral theory, we conclude that much, perhaps most, of this research is merely relevant to ethics rather than being part of it; in particular, the role to be played by the sociology of ethics, and by research into public attitudes on moral issues, is extremely limited.

2. The "Fact-Value Gap"

One of the principal reasons given for casting doubt on the relevance of empirical data to ethical conclusions is the claim that descriptive facts and values seem to be quite different kinds of things. In one version of this claim, facts (for example about the widespread political use of torture) are real and objectively there, so that we can make true statements about them, whereas whatever values (for example the wrongness of torture) are, they are not thought to be like *that*. This difference is sometimes called the "fact-value gap," the metaphor of a gap being used to capture the idea that this difference in kind is a profound one that cannot easily be bridged. In particular, the gap between fact and value prevents from us inferring evaluative statements (statements about right and wrong, good and bad) from purely descriptive premises. So, for example, no amount of empirical information about intractable pain in some terminally ill patients can *by itself* allow us to infer that euthanasia is right, for the gap between the descriptive information and the evaluative conclusion prevents any such inference from being valid. Unless we have something like a moral principle saying that killing the innocent is sometimes morally permissible, the inference just will not go through. And this failure of inference may be thought to cast doubt upon the relevance of empirical data to *any* ethical conclusions, including bioethical ones, since such data can never settle ethical debates.

But this further thought is open to two objections. First, it is not warranted by the existence of a fact-value gap, since there may be ways of bridging the gap that will at least allow empirical evidence to be relevant to ethical issues, even if it cannot settle them on its own. As we saw above, the presence of a bridging principle about which actions are morally permissible, or even obligatory, can do this work. And second, the very existence of a fact-value gap of the traditional kind, understood as a profound metaphysical difference between facts and values, is itself highly debatable.

On the traditional account of the fact-value gap, facts are real and describable in true statements, whereas values are subjective, and evaluative statements are not capable of truth or falsity at all. But even on this account, it is still possible for empirical data to play a significant role in ethical debate. If ethical statements are just expressions of our attitudes toward different features of the world, or are effectively prescriptions for action based on those attitudes, then we need the empirical data to tell us which features of the world are actually present. If we have the attitude of approval toward general happiness, let us say, or perhaps on the basis of that attitude prescribe actions which tend to promote it, then we need to know which actions do actually promote happiness. So on this (broadly non-cognitivist) understanding of morality, empirical data will be essential to the formation of our moral views, since they will tell us what features are present for our approval or disapproval. Even though they cannot settle moral issues all by themselves—since we still have to bring our attitudes to bear on them to generate an evaluation—the data are still relevant to our moral conclusions.

However, this traditional understanding of the fact-value gap is by no means the only one available. Those who think that value statements are capable of truth and falsity, so that some amount of objectivity is a feature of the moral domain, will regard the difference between facts and values as more like the difference between physical facts and biological facts, where the latter are understood as a subset of the former. Values, that is, are to be seen as a kind of fact, so that the contrast is between evaluative facts and descriptive facts. (This view is perfectly compatible with there still being an is-ought gap.[3]) The gap here is no longer so deep and unbridgeable; since values and empirical data now turn out to be different kinds of fact, the way is open for a closer relationship between them.

There are other reasons to think that that relationship is quite close. First, the existence of "thick" ethical concepts,[4] such as courage or kindness or cruelty, shows that sometimes empirical and evaluative facts are so intertwined that they cannot be disentangled. A judgment that somebody is courageous carries empirical and evaluative content, but these are not conceptually separable—we cannot pick out the empirical facts about who is courageous without having a firm grasp of the kind of evaluation that is involved here.[5] And when we are formulating our scientific theories, quite separately from any considerations to do with morality, we nonetheless find that values are an essential part of the process. This is because epistemic values such as simplicity and coherence are an indispensable element in theory choice: we use them to select the best of a competing range of theories, and consequently they are inextricably involved in establishing just what the facts are.[6] So values are sometimes involved in establishing what the empirical facts are, and it would not be entirely surprising if the reverse were also true.

There is also another important theoretical reason why we might expect empirical facts to play an important part in ethical debates. A notable feature (and for some, a defining feature) of morality is that there is something universal about our moral judgments. If (for example) it is wrong for one person deliberately to kill innocent civilians, then it is wrong for *anyone* in relevantly similarly circumstances deliberately to kill innocent civilians; such actions are wrong *in virtue of* being the deliberate killing of innocents. (This is to say that moral properties supervene upon non-moral ones.[7]) But this means that in some sense the empirical facts fix the moral facts, so that they are a genuine part of the ethical debate. Just *which* empirical facts play this role, in which circumstances, is itself disputed, and much will depend on which normative ethical theory turns out to be the most successful one.

But in a given situation, some empirical facts will be able to play this fixing or determining role, whereas others will not, although they may still be relevant to how the debate goes. So, for example, the facts about how much pain a particular treatment will alleviate may be genuinely part of the ethical debate about whether it ought to be adopted, because these facts may (help to) determine the rightness of that decision. By contrast, facts about public faith (or lack of it) in the treatment may not be actually *part* of that debate, even though they may have some *relevance* to it (for example they may be relevant to the speed with which the treatment should be adopted, or to how the decision to do so should be publicly presented).

This aspect of morality, that moral features of a situation or action are present in virtue of the presence of some non-moral properties, so that the non-moral properties *determine* the moral ones, is a crucial one for our argument. This is what enables us to draw an important distinction, between empirical facts that are part of a particular ethical debate because they help determine the rightness (or wrongness) of what is to be done, and empirical facts that are merely relevant to the debate, playing a more tangential role. How this distinction is to be run will vary from case to case. But as a general point, although there is no reason to think we must keep empirical data at arm's length when we are doing ethics, some empirical information is more equal than others, so to speak, and we may not want to give a full entry-ticket to everything that on the face of it appears germane.

Large claims have been made concerning the centrality to ethics of some kinds of empirical data, both from the natural sciences and from the social sciences. Perhaps the most notable claim has been made for data from evolutionary psychology and biology, especially concerning behavior that promotes survival and reproduction. Some sociobiologists have suggested that such data are enough to settle major ethical issues,[8] so that if altruism, for example, can be shown to promote survival and reproduction, then we have found a justification for engaging in altruistic behavior. But since we have no reason to believe that altruistic actions are right in virtue of promoting survival and reproduction, then even if facts about the promotion of survival and reproduction turn out to be relevant to ethical debates, we do not thereby have reason to think they are part of ethics, or to think that they can by themselves provide a justification for altruistic behavior.

Other data from the sciences are sometimes presented as part of ethics, and in subsequent sections we consider some of these. Our prime concern is the role of social science in bioethics. However, we start by taking a brief look at the natural sciences.

3. The Role of Natural Science

Obviously, the morality of an action or policy will often depend partly upon the facts of natural science: especially, in the case of bioethics, biological facts. (For example, in reproductive medicine, evidence about the health effects of sperm sorting, pre-implantation genetic diagnosis (PGD), in vitro fertilization (IVF), intracytoplasmic sperm injection (ICSI), and suchlike on resultant children is relevant to the question of whether such practices should be prohibited.) It would however be extremely odd to call natural science research "ethics," even though its findings are undoubtedly relevant to ethics. This is hardly surprising since, if we allowed scientific research into the likely consequences of our actions to count as ethics, then the floodgates would be open and almost *all* research would or could be ethics research (because almost all research can, in particular circumstances, be relevant to ethics).

Our second point about natural science (one which follows from some of the theoretical considerations discussed earlier) is that scientific research alone is never sufficient to settle an ethical question. Returning to the reproductive medicine case mentioned above, for example, both sides in this debate ("restrictive" and "permissive") might agree that child welfare will be adversely affected by the use of a particular technology, but nonetheless disagree about whether this is sufficient to justify prohibition—perhaps because there is an underlying moral or philosophical dispute about the significance of "the non-identity problem," or about the importance of parental autonomy.[9] In cases like these, gathering further biological or psychological evidence about the welfare of future children will not move the debate forwards, since what is at issue is a moral or philosophical matter, not an empirical one. Even if we knew everything that there was to know about child welfare, the dispute would persist.

We conclude, then, first that natural science is not a part of ethics, even though its results are often relevant to ethics, and second that natural science research alone is never sufficient to settle an ethical question.

4. Social Science: Some Preliminaries

We noted earlier that research into the likely consequences of our actions is obviously relevant to ethics. As Robert Zussman puts it, "A good deal of medical ethics is based on consequentialist claims that social scientists are well equipped to deal with."[10] This is the main way in which social science can contribute to bioethics, since knowing what the social consequences would be if we did x will often be a crucial part of the moral case for or against doing x. To take a straightforward example, Bob Brecher, arguing against commercial surrogacy, claims that "a pool of surrogates could well be created on the model of working class prostitution; women would come to be imported from poor countries for the purpose of serving as surrogates…."[11]

In order fully to assess Brecher's moral argument, we would need social and economic data to confirm or falsify what he says about the likelihood of importing surrogates "from poor countries." More generally, the same goes for many of the slippery slope arguments that find their way into almost every bioethical debate. Insofar as these are empirical "slope" arguments, appealing to the harmful social consequences of adopting a certain policy, ethics can clearly benefit from the work of social scientists, whose job it is to provide empirical evidence for or against such assertions.

Does anything follow from the fact that sociological research into the likely consequences of our actions is (or should be) of interest to ethicists? Probably not, or not much. For, as we saw earlier, mere relevance to ethics is not enough to make something part of ethics, and the role of social science just sketched is not fundamentally different from that of natural science, because both simply deliver information about the effects of our actions. However, several writers have expressed dissatisfaction with this "usual account of moral reasoning" according to which

> social science is often seen as able to provide "just the facts," while philosophy attends to moral values and conceptual clarity and builds formally valid arguments.[12]

Mairi Levitt describes this as "the traditional view of bioethics as moral philosophy," according to which:

> sociologists are junior technicians in the bioethical enterprise rather than equal partners. Where bioethics is concerned with normative ethics, setting out what ought to be done, if sociologists are required at all they will only be useful to provide background data. The philosopher may select from these data, but any empirical research will always be subordinate to moral reasoning.[13]

Erica Haimes, meanwhile, talks of "the over-simplistic division between normative and descriptive ethics (that assigns the social sciences the 'handmaiden' role of simply providing the 'facts')."[14] So to dismiss social science at this stage as "not part of ethics" (or as merely its "handmaiden") would perhaps be too hasty, since there are other possible roles that it might occupy. In the next few sections, we explore these, along with some arguments for the view that its role in ethics is central rather than peripheral.

5. The Sociology of Ethics

In the previous section, we were thinking mainly of social science as delivering information about the effects on society of our actions and policies. A rather different social science endeavor is the sociology of ethics. This comes in two main forms. First, there are studies of the behavior of ethicists.

Second, there is public attitudes research, which studies the moral views of the general public (or some appropriate subset thereof).

Haimes suggests a reason why we should take the first ("the sociology of ethicists") seriously:

> whilst there is still a legitimate case to be made for seeing ethics as an abstract formal discipline, distanced from matters of actual social practice, it is not possible to posit the same view of ethicists themselves. As individual and collective practitioners of their discipline, however varied in their approaches and interests, they are members of professional and other social groupings and are thus subject to the influences of, and in turn influence, broader social changes and developments.[15]

We would not disagree with what Haimes says here, since clearly ethicists affect and are affected by social phenomena. However, we would question whether much follows from this. For we could say pretty much the same about *any* academic subject (or any practice). And so Haimes's claim does not entail the view that the "sociology of ethicists" is (or ought to be) part of ethics. After all, in most areas, we would not say that the sociology of a subject was part of that subject: for example the sociology of physics is not itself physics. So, while acknowledging that it is useful for ethicists to know about the sociology of their subject, we doubt that that gives us reason to view sociology as an integral part of ethics.

A second (stronger) reason for rejecting the "sociology as part of ethics" view is that knowing about the sociology of academic ethics will not (except in quite unusual cases) provide us with reasons to accept or reject ethical arguments. This is because the soundness of an argument is separable from its origins. So (for example) discovering that 90% of bioethicists were white male Catholics would not, in and of itself, tell us anything about the quality of these bioethicists' arguments against procreative autonomy. This sociological fact would make us suspicious of their arguments (and rightly so), and make us subject them to more careful scrutiny than usual (not least because we would suspect them of bias). But if the arguments are sound then they are sound no matter who propounds them. Another way of making essentially the same point would be to say that to reject (or accept) an ethical argument on sociological grounds (for example, because of facts about the people who put it forward) would be fallaciously to use an *ad hominem* move, defined by Nigel Warburton as "attacking the character of the person with whom you are arguing rather than finding fault with his or her argument."[16]

6. Public Attitudes Research

> 1,000 people were asked whether Einstein, Jesus, Mozart, or Elvis Presley should be cloned for the benefit of mankind. 22% voted for Einstein compared with just 12% who thought Jesus should be cloned. Mozart was chosen by 8% and Elvis by 7%. A total of 61% said none of the four should be cloned, and 5% said they did not know. Some of those questioned chose more than one name. 10% of men agreed humans should be cloned, compared with 7% of women.[17]

The rest of our chapter looks at *public attitudes research*, by which we mean research into what "the public" thinks about ethical issues. Such research can take several forms, ranging from more or less crude quantitative surveys (like the one quoted above) through to more subtle ethnographic and qualitative work.[18] Obviously, public attitudes research can sometimes be relevant to bioethics in the same way that natural science research is. But in what follows we question the view that it is any more important (or any more "ethics") than natural science research, along with the view that it is part of (as opposed to merely relevant to) bioethics.

In discussions about the role of public attitudes research, philosophers often accuse sociologists of being relativists, while the sociologists return the favor by accusing the philosophers of not being relativistic enough![19] For this reason, we'll start our examination of public attitudes research with some thoughts about relativism.

The relevant relativism for our purposes is moral relativism: more specifically, metaethical relativism, which says (roughly) that there is no single true or most justified morality and that moral propositions are true—insofar as they are true at all—just in virtue of their conforming to the relevant society's attitudes or conventions. This view should be carefully distinguished from, and definitely is not entailed by, descriptive relativism, the view that there is, as a matter of fact, extensive cross-cultural and interpersonal diversity in moral attitudes and opinions. So, according to moral relativism, a particular practice—say, sex between adults and children—may be "wrong-for-us" (for example the population of England) because we generally have negative attitudes to such relationships, but at the same time "right-for-them" (some other society) because in "their" society sex between adults and children is generally approved of.

Relativism of this sort has several implications for ethics but, for our present purposes, the main one is methodological. For if, as relativism tells us, what makes propositions such as "x is wrong" true (or "true for S," where S is a relevant social group) is the fact that "x is wrong" is endorsed by most members of the relevant community, then we can find out the answer to all ethical questions just by surveying people and finding out what they think. So, if relativism is true, then bioethics should be little more than a branch of sociology. For sociologists could (in principle) give us the answer to ethics questions such as "is cloning wrong?" just by surveying people and finding out what they think about cloning. If people generally like cloning, then it is permissible or good. If they do not, then it is wrong.[20]

Our view is that ethics is not a branch of sociology and that, on the contrary, sociology is peripheral to ethics. Given what we have just said, crucial to this view is the rejection of metaethical relativism. This is not the place to attempt a thoroughgoing refutation, but we can at least briefly outline our principal reasons for dismissing it.

One major defect in the theory is the uncritical identification of "might" (majority opinion or social convention) with "right" (what people really ought to do). For while public opinion should sometimes be taken into account when framing policy, there is no necessary connection between what "society thinks" about any given issue and the moral truth of the matter. In other words, it is possible for "society to think" that cloning is immoral even if there is nothing wrong with it. Or, to employ more telling (if rather clichéd) examples, it would be possible for a "society to think" that sex between adults and children, genocide, and torturing kittens were all morally permissible, even if really such practices were wrong.

A second unattractive feature (one closely related to the first) is that relativism commits us, as ethicists, to being deeply conservative, or at least conservative with respect to the present conventions and practices of our own society. This is because, if relativism were true, we could simply "read off" the answers to moral questions from public opinion and because there would be no standpoint from which to criticize prevailing views on moral matters. This is interesting because, in conversation with us, sociologists have sometimes presented moral relativism as a politically radical position, whereas in fact it is the opposite.

If we reject moral relativism then we are left with a puzzle about what sociology's proper role within bioethics could be. For if it is not legitimate to argue directly from (say) "90% of people disapprove of x" to either "x is wrong" or "x should be banned," then it is not clear why ethicists should care about the fact that "90% of people disapprove of x."

7. Consultation Exercises

> Almost all publicly funded ethics research of the sort undertaken or commissioned by ethics committees or commissions takes it as axiomatic that some attempt to discover what people think about the issues under consideration is part of the remit. But the point and purpose of obtaining this information is seldom clear.[21]

A possible rationale for undertaking and taking seriously public attitudes research is as part of a consultation process. A relevant example here is the

Human Fertilization and Embryology Authority's recent consultation entitled *Sex Selection: Choice and Responsibility in Human Reproduction.*[22] Under the heading "What is the Purpose of this Consultation?" the HFEA says:

> In January [2002] we commissioned two independent reports, one on the range, safety and reliability of the techniques currently available for sex selection, and the other on the social and ethical considerations that relate to them. In June [2002] qualitative market research involving several discussion groups was conducted into public attitudes towards sex selection in the UK and to support this, we have commissioned further quantitative research on this subject.[23]
>
> The purpose of this consultation document is … to seek the views of the public concerning under what circumstances sex selection should be avail-able to those seeking treatment and whether any new legal provisions should be put in place to regulate it ….[24]

The HFEA's information gathering process contains several distinct elements.

- An expert report analyzing and summarizing extant medical research.
- An expert report on "the social and ethical considerations."
- Responses to a consultation document.
- Specially commissioned primary empirical research using social science ("market research") techniques, both qualitative and quantitative.

It is worth paying some attention to what exactly the role of each element is (or should be). (1) appears reasonably unproblematic and would be covered by what we said earlier about the position of natural science research in bioethics. More or less the same goes for (2), although the issue of who gets to count as an expert on "ethical and social" matters may be contentious. (3) differs from the other elements because it is not really research at all—except (trivially) insofar as it is research into what happens when the HFEA releases a consultation document on sex selection. It is not public attitudes research, because there is no reason to believe that the responses will be representative. Indeed, the results generated by these processes are often quite unrepresentative, because they attract mass responses from pressure groups. (A good example of this problem is described in the *Brazier Report* on surrogacy.[25])

Consultation processes, then, are not reliable guides to "current public and professional attitudes," and filtering needs to be used to screen out the distortions created not only by pressure groups, but also by the obvious fact that most ordinary people (those without a special personal interest) have neither the time nor the inclination to respond to official consultations on reproductive technology and suchlike. This filtering cannot (or should not) be done *a priori* and ought to be based on independent social science research. But if such research already exists, then why is the consultation process necessary? And, more generally, given that consultation exercises like these do not deliver trustworthy information about public attitudes, what is their real purpose?

There appear to be two realistic possibilities. One is that consultation exercises are not research tools at all, but instead part of a democratic process. This may well be true and, if it is, then while consultation exercises will have a point, their point will not have anything to do with public attitudes research, since consultation exercises will not be research, any more than general elections are research. A second possibility is that the job of a consultation exercise is to trawl for arguments that can later be subjected to critical assessment by ethicists (and relevant others). This sounds like what the HFEA has in mind when it says:

> We would especially welcome more substantial contributions from anyone who has a strong interest in this subject. The HFEA intends to *listen carefully to all the arguments* put forward.[26]

The idea appears to be that experts and informed "lay" people will donate arguments for assessment by the HFEA experts. If this is the point of consultation exercises then they may well have a role in ethics, albeit a minor one, because they are a source of moral arguments (or elements thereof). They provide the "raw material" out of which moral philosophers (and others) can fashion coherent sets of policies and principles.

Let us turn now to the part of the HFEA's process that is explicitly labeled social science ("market") research. The point of the market research in this con-sultation is unclear, especially if we keep in mind the earlier rejection of moral relativism and the fact that this is supposed to be *research*, not a referendum on sex selection. Another way of getting at the problem is to ask: what if it turns out that 80% of people are against sex selection (except for "medical" reasons), but that the arguments for this majority view are all unsound? If we are doing ethics (as opposed to merely trying to arrive at a political compromise), then the arguments (or lack thereof) must prevail over the views of the 80%, and this might make us wonder why we bothered to spend money on the market research in the first place.

We conclude then that the existence of official consultation processes does not in any way bolster the position of public attitudes research within bioethics. Our reasons are first that much of what might be seen as public attitudes research within the consultation process is either unreliable or not research at all, and second, for policymakers, the *arguments* must prevail over the views of the majority where the two come into conflict (so rendering public attitudes research irrelevant, except insofar as it performs the peripheral "handmaiden" or "argument trawling" roles discussed earlier).

8. Public Attitudes Research and Psychological Harm

As we have already suggested, a valid use of public attitudes research (within the "handmaiden" paradigm) is to discover whether a proposed policy will have harmful psychological or social effects. We might argue, for example, that if 80% of adults were frightened by the prospect of human reproductive cloning, then we would have a reason for banning cloning, since large numbers of people would sleep easier in their beds knowing that an "attack of the clones" had been rendered less likely by restrictive laws. On this view, banning cloning could be justified by reference to the psychological harm it causes.

On the face of it, this use of public attitudes research looks just like the legitimate use of natural science research discussed earlier, since both simply warn us about the harmful effects of our actions. However, one complication is that some forms of psychological harm are caused by attitudes that are apt for rational assessment. It is widely accepted, even by liberals, that if a practice is substantially harmful to innocent third parties then there is a *prima facie* case for banning it. However, in order to be plausible, this "harm principle" must be restricted so that only some types of harm are allowed to count. In particular, we must exclude psychological harm that would not have occurred were it not for the unreasonable beliefs of the "victim." In other words, it would be wrong to ban something just because people were unreasonably afraid of or distressed or repulsed by it: for example, if either their moral beliefs (for example "cloning violates human dignity") or their non-moral beliefs (for example "if cloning is permitted then the world will be overrun by Hitler replicants") were unreasonable.

What if, for example, a majority of the population was unreasonably repulsed by the existence of churches and by the existence of gay sex? Would this provide a good reason to ban them? We would (and should) answer "definitely not," even if people really were psychologically harmed by the presence of these things. Of course, other State measures to prevent the psychological harm might be warranted—most obviously, a public education campaign to stop people from having such unreasonable views. But to impose bans would be to pander to people's irrational fears and feelings, and would be an unfair violation of the rights of gay people and Christians.[27] (We should add that not all irrational fears are unreasonable, as we use the term—for example, it would probably be wrong to call most pathological fear unreasonable.)

It is not hard to see how similar thoughts apply to less exotic examples, especially for our purposes public attitudes to issues in bioethics. Take the following example of social science research, described by Haimes:

> Edwards … provides valuable insight into how ordinary people, with no direct involvement with assisted conception, think about … ethical and social issues. In her ethnographic study of "Alltown," she discovered that residents identified three related sets of dangers with these practices: psychological (in terms of worrying about the effects on the children conceived), biological (in terms of the risks of incest which was used as a "conceptual brake. . . a boundary, a limit which ought not to be traversed") and relational (the impact of reproductive technologies on wider social relationships).[28]

We do not doubt that Edwards's research is interesting and worthwhile. What is more questionable, though, is its ability to contribute to ethics. This is principally because of the reasonableness constraint just discussed. Edwards's "ordinary people" offer three possible objections to reproductive technology: the welfare of children created, concerns about "incest" (or quasi-incestuous reproductive practices), and effects "on wider social relationships." Does this tell us anything about the bioethical issues in question? For several interconnected reasons, probably not.

First, ethicists do not usually need social science research to tell them about the existence of moral arguments—and, as it happens, the objections cited by Edwards are precisely the kinds of things already widely discussed by moral philosophers. It is probable then that, in most cases, these philosophers will be capable of generating the relevant arguments for themselves (which is, after all, what they do best) without relying on public attitudes research to do it for them. (We do not deny, though, that there will be a small number of cases in which the ethicists are incapable of coming up with the arguments themselves.)

Second, because of the reasonableness constraint, knowing that many people endorse these three objections does not matter much for the purposes of ethics and policy. Either these objections are reasonable or they are not. If they are reasonable, then this is something that bioethics could in principle discover without knowing that the objections are widely subscribed to: that is, without the public attitudes research. But if, like being repulsed by the existence of churches, the objections are unreasonable then they should be disregarded, or at least should not directly influence ethics or policy. They may however influence it indirectly by prompting more education spending, or by providing an empirical premise in a pragmatic policy argument—for example "we had better not allow x, or there will be rioting."

9. Conclusion

During the first few sections of the chapter, we saw that the general theoretical case for keeping empirical evidence out of ethics is weak, and that an ethics that disregards the empirical facts will be seriously impoverished. It does not however follow from this that all kinds of empirical data are able to enter equally into ethical debate and, with this in mind, we spent most of the rest of the chapter examining the proper place of sociological evidence within academic bioethics. Our aim was not to criticize social scientists or to argue that bioethicists should refuse to work with or ignore them. On the contrary, we agree with Levitt that:

> Together philosophical and sociological bioethics can widen the bioethical perspective by setting an issue or problem in its historical, social, cultural, and political context.[29]

However, we have defended the view that the function of the social sciences is what Haimes terms the "'handmaiden' role of providing the 'facts,'" along with the view that sociology is (therefore) peripheral rather than central to bioethics—like natural science, a mere supplier of empirical premises which can be "plugged in" to bioethical arguments.

NOTES

1. See the allegory of the cave, Plato, *The Republic*, trans. H. D. P. Lee (Harmond-sworth: Penguin Books, 1972), VII 514a–521b

2. Aristotle, *Nicomachean Ethics*, trans. W. D. Ross, revised by J. L.Ackrill and J. O. Urmson (Oxford: Oxford University Press, 1980), p. 160.

3. See David Wiggins, "Truth, Invention, and the Meaning of Life," *Proceedings of the British Academy*, 62 (1976), pp. 331–378.

4. See Bernard Williams, *Ethics and the Limits of Philosophy* (London: Fontana Press, 1985).

5. See John McDowell, "Non-Cognitivism and Rule-Following," *Wittgenstein: To Follow a Rule*, ed. Steven H. Holtzmann and Christopher M. Leich (London, Routledge and Kegan Paul, 1981).

6. See Hilary Putnam, "The Collapse of the Fact-Value Dichotomy," *The Collapse of the Fact-Value Dichotomy and Other Essays* (Cambridge, MA: Harvard University Press, 2002).

7. See Richard Hare, *The Language of Morals* (Oxford: Oxford University Press, 1952).

8. Michael Ruse and Edward Wilson, "Moral Philosophy as Applied Science," *Philosophy*, 61:236 (April 1986), pp. 173–192.

9. David McCarthy, "Why Sex Selection Should be Legal," *Journal of Medical Ethics*, 27:5 (October 2001), p. 304. See also: Robert Boyle and Julian Savulescu, "Ethics of Using Preimplantation Genetic Diagnosis to Select a Stem Cell Donor for an Existing Person," *British Medical Journal*, 323:7323 (24 November 2001), p. 1242.

10. Robert Zussman, "The Contributions of Sociology to Medical Ethics," *Hastings Center Report*, 30:1 (January–February 2000), p. 9.

11. Robert Brecher, "Surrogacy, Liberal Individualism and the Moral Climate," *Moral Philosophy and Contemporary Problems*, ed. J. D. G. Evans (Cambridge: Cambridge University Press, 1987), p. 195.

12. James Lindemann Nelson, "Moral Teachings from Unexpected Quarters: Lessons for Bioethics from the Social Sciences and Managed Care," *Hastings Center Report*, 30:1 (January–February 2000), p. 12.

13. Mairi Levitt, "Better Together? Sociological and Philosophical Perspectives on Bioethics," *Scratching the Surface of Bioethics*, ed. Matti Häyry and Tuija Takala (Amsterdam: Rodopi, 2003), p. 11. See also Søren Holm, *Ethical Problems in Clinical Practice* (Manchester: Manchester University Press, 1997), pp. 23–39; Zussman, "The Contributions of Sociology to Medical Ethics," p. 9.

14. Erica Haimes, "What Can the Social Sciences Contribute to the Study of Ethics? Theoretical, Empirical, and Substantive Considerations," *Bioethics*, 16:2 (April 2002), p. 89.

15. Haimes, "What Can the Social Sciences Contribute to the Study of Ethics?," pp. 92–3.

16 . Nigel Warburton, *Thinking from A to Z* (London: Routledge, 2nd ed., 2000), p. 70.

17. Ananova (www.ananova.com), "Clone Einstein Not Jesus," 28 January 2003.

18. For a useful overview see *Methods in Medical Ethics*, ed. Jeremy Sugarman and Daniel P. Sulmasy (Washington, DC: Georgetown University Press, 2001), pp. 146–191.

19. Levitt, "Better Together?," p. 12.

20. See Eve Garrard and Stephen Wilkinson, "Does Bioethics Need Moral Theory?," *Scratching the Surface of Bioethics*, ed. Matti Häyry and Tuija Takala (Amsterdam: Rodopi, 2003), pp. 35–45.

21. John Harris, "Introduction: The Scope and Importance of Bioethics," *Bioethics*, ed. John Harris (Oxford: Oxford University Press, 2001), pp. 7–8.

22. The Human Fertilisation and Embryology Association (HFEA), *Sex Selection: Choice and Responsibility in Human Reproduction*, www.hfea.gov.uk, 2002.

23. The HFEA, *Sex Selection*, p. 5.

24. The HFEA , *Sex Selection*, p. 6.

25. Margaret Brazier, Alastair Campbell, and Susan Golombok, *Surrogacy: Review for Health Ministers of Current Arrangements for Payments and Regulation* (London: The Stationery Office, 1998).

26. The HFEA, *Sex Selection*, p. 6 (our emphasis).

27. See Sally Sheldon and Stephen Wilkinson, "Female Genital Mutilation and Cosmetic Surgery: Regulating Non-Therapeutic Body Modification," *Bioethics*, 12:4 (October 1998), pp. 263–285.

28. Haimes, "What Can the Social Sciences Contribute to the Study of Ethics?," p. 103.

29. Levitt, "Better Together?," p. 17.

Eight

INFORMED CONSENT: BIOETHICAL IDEAL AND EMPIRICAL REALITY

Angus Dawson

1. Introduction

It is now almost universally held that patients undergoing clinical encounters or participating in medical research are required to give an informed consent. The trend to argue that this is so began in earnest in the bioethics literature thirty years ago and has now grown to encompass virtually all professional, national, and international bodies with any role in governance issues in relation to both research and clinical medicine. (For example, the Nuremberg Code[1] and the Helsinki Declaration[2] were formulated with the intention of protecting research subjects from abuse, and both documents give prominence to recognizable forms of informed consent. They both specifically identify information about the nature of the research, any risks and benefits, and details about the methodology as being of central concern. Leading policy documents by the United Kingdom's Department of Health,[3] the British Medical Association,[4] and the General Medical Council[5] all suggest informed consent should now be considered a routine aspect of clinical practice as well as of research.)

However, despite this consensus about the need for informed consent there has been a series of papers, going back nearly as far as the existence of the concept itself, suggesting that there are serious problems in attempting to turn this laudable ideal into reality. This research seems to suggest that there are real and persistent problems in gaining an informed consent amongst at least a subset of each of the groups studied. Despite this literature, the noisy advocacy in favor of informed consent has continued to grow. This chapter is a review of the empirical evidence that suggests that gaining an informed consent is difficult or impossible, at least with these subgroups. I argue that this evidence is too consistent and too important to be ignored, and that supporters of the concept of informed consent need to address the issues that are raised by these studies: informed consent as a bioethical ideal needs to face up to empirical reality.

2. What is "Informed Consent?"

Many different definitions of "informed consent" have been proposed. For example, Tom Beauchamp and James Childress offer a very full analysis of the "elements" of the concept. They break it down into seven different components: competence, voluntariness, disclosure of information, recommendation of a plan, understanding, a decision, and authorization of the relevant action.[6] In contrast, Bernard Gert, Charles M. Culver, and K. Danner Clouser use the term "valid consent"[7] in preference to "informed consent," and they focus only on three key "criteria" as follows: adequate information provision for the patient, non-coercion of the patient, and assessment of the patient as being competent. Some commentators, such as Stephen Wear,[8] seem content to give up on an analysis of the concept altogether and opt for a more pragmatic account instead: one containing a range of variables to be combined in different ways depending upon the situation. Despite this skepticism about picking out the concept, his discussion makes clear that there is still enough common ground between these different accounts to be sure that they are all talking about the same thing.

I will use the term "informed consent" in this chapter, as this is the most widely used and understood term in relation to the issue under consideration. I will, however, focus on the three key components as suggested by Gert and his collaborators. We can frame these "criteria" as questions as follows: Is the person competent? Is the decision free from influence or coercion? Was the relevant information provided, and did it form the basis of the decision? I will discuss each of these in turn. This section attempts to describe why each issue is considered to be an essential element of informed consent.

A. Competence

Being competent or having capacity is a necessary ability for understanding the relevant information about different possible interventions, and for making the decision about which option to adopt. Exactly what competence involves, and how it is to be determined, has been subject to much debate since the publication of Allen E. Buchanan and Dan W. Brock's *Deciding for Others*.[9] Buchanan and Brock argue that competence should be viewed as being related to the particular decision to be made and to the degree of risk of harm attached to the possible outcome of that decision. On this view, riskier decisions require a greater degree of competence. This approach has been both challenged and defended in the bioethics literature.[10] Whatever the correct account of competence, it is vital that a clear definition is given by the defenders of informed consent so that the competent and incompetent can be clearly distinguished. This is held to be necessary so that we can respect the autonomy of the competent individuals: they will be able to make their own decisions and are presumed to be capable of giving an informed consent. However, clear arrangements will also have to be in place for decision-making in relation to incompetent patients. This might involve judgments about what is in an individual's best interests or a role for advance directives or proxy decision makers.[11]

B. Free Decision

The reason to believe that this is an important element of informed consent is that the decision reached by the individual must be her own, free from the influence, manipulation, or coercion of all other parties. This element might be breached not just through attempted persuasion, but also through deception or the manipulation of information to try to obtain a particular end. This type of influence need not be intentional, as indirect influence might well just follow from certain types of relationship (for example, doctor-patient relationships, family relationships, and so on). Where this is a potential danger, the supporter of informed consent will argue that care should be taken to ensure that indirect influence does not occur.

C. Information Provision and Understanding

This is the core element in any account of informed consent, as both competence and the ability to make a free choice might be held to be pre-conditions for an informed consent rather than, strictly speaking, part of the consent itself. However, an informed consent cannot be given without the provision of the relevant information, and without that information being understood by the patient. Information will be relevant in relation to diagnosis, prognosis, the nature and purpose of the available alternative interventions, and the associated risks and benefits of each option. It is also important to include reference to the consequences of non-treatment. It has long been recognized that different people have different abilities to understand such information, and different amounts of pre-existing knowledge to draw upon for deliberation.

However, in response it has been argued that physicians can use other methods to try to ensure that the patient has understood the information. For example, an opportunity might be explicitly given for questions, or perhaps the patient could be seen on a number of different occasions (at least in a non-emergency situation). It is also often pointed out that a patient might be shy, over-awed, in pain, or afraid given the nature of the clinical encounter. Can the information be given in such a way that it is not overwhelming? Does it need to be repeated? For these reasons, the supporters of informed consent place great importance upon the need for good communication skills. They will argue that the ideal system would be one in which doctors respond to the individual abilities and wishes of the patient, but in which essentially all competent patients are assumed to give either an informed consent or autonomously waive their right to do so. For the rest of this chapter I will focus only on the issue of information giving and assume that the other two components (voluntariness and competence) are unproblematic.

3. Informed Consent as Bioethical Ideal

So far, then, I have suggested that informed consent consists of a free decision made by a competent person on the basis of relevant information, and that the demand for physicians to gain such a consent is widely believed to be a moral requirement. Now that we are clear about what counts as an informed consent, we can move onto the next question: why should we seek it? There are two main ethical justifications for seeking an informed consent given in the literature. The most common one is to appeal to auto-nomy or self-determination, but Brock[12] reminds us that it is also possible to provide a justification by appealing to the role that informed consent might play within an account of patient well-being. I will briefly consider both possibilities here.

Autonomy is a difficult concept to define, but can be roughly characterized as involving the control or direction of the decisions and actions of an individual by that particular individual herself. This means that there may be both an internal (or psychological) aspect and an external (or political) aspect. The individual is autonomous in the "internal" sense when she is free to choose what she wants, and other things, such as addictions, do not influence her choices. She is autonomous in the "external" sense when she is able to act freely because she is not physically restrained or imprisoned, and so on. The appeal of autonomy for the justification of informed consent is to general beliefs about the rights of the individual to control or govern what happens to her own body. It is held by the supporters of the pro-autonomy view that this is the best way of avoiding other people making decisions on our behalf. The classic statement of this principle is to be found in John Stuart Mill's *On Liberty*:

> [T]he only purpose for which power can be rightfully exercised over any member of a civilised community, against his will, is to prevent harm to others. His own good, either physical or moral, is not sufficient warrant. He cannot rightfully be compelled to do or forbear because it will be better for him to do so, because it will make him happier, because in the opinion of others, to do so would be wise or even right.[13]

Any attempt to interfere in such decision-making in relation to the relevant individual runs the risk of the accusation of paternalism. It is worth noting that although the term "paternalism" is often invoked in such contexts, it is frequently used pejoratively as though the mere description of an act in this way were enough to explain and justify its wrongness. There is no reason to think this, of course, unless we wish to stipulate that paternalism is simply to have this particular (condemnatory) meaning. Situations where an informed consent is not sought might well be paternalistic but this, on its own, does not mean that they are wrong.[14] The argument for seeking informed consent is that this is more likely to allow genuine autonomous participation by the individuals themselves. (The appeal of such autonomous participation may, in turn, be justified through an appeal to an ethical theory such as consequentialism, deontology, rights theory, or a principle such as self-ownership.) It is certainly the case that autonomy-based justifications of informed consent gain strong support through the fact that whenever surveys are conducted about whether patients want to give such consent to medical procedures, a clear majority answer that they do.[15]

The standard view, then, is that informed consent is vital as a means of both ensuring and promoting the autonomy or self-determination of medical patients. Much recent discussion of issues in healthcare ethics proceeds as though it is autonomy or self-determination that is the core value to be promoted within medicine, and seeking informed consent is one of the central methods by which this is to be achieved. (These ethical arguments can be strengthened by looking at some of the historical reasons for the growth of interest in informed consent. This has emerged as a response to historical events in relation to medical research, and the development of legal protection for the rights of individuals to be informed about their treatment and the research they participate in.[16]) However, there is a strong counter-argument to this, which is that autonomy is only one of many moral considerations, and other factors such as beneficence need to be given their relevant weighting in the moral judgment to be made. This view might be supported by the thought that any plausible moral theory (such as Rossian deontology, many forms of consequentialism, the four principles, and so on) will be pluralist and want to trade off different values against each other, with different ones taking priority depending upon the circumstances.

The second possible way of justifying an appeal to informed consent is to look toward patient well-being. The idea here is that involving the patient in the consent process might well increase patient well-being or welfare because she is going to be better informed, more involved in the decision-making, her autonomy is respected, and she is less likely to feel anxious as possibilities about the future are explained. Such a justification is much broader than the appeal to autonomy. On this view, of course, autonomy might be a component of well-being, but other factors will also be held to contribute toward the individual's good.

There appear, then, to be strong ethical arguments in favor of seeking informed consent, as both autonomy and well-being are very important moral considerations. Let us accept, at least for the purposes of this chapter, that the moral case in favor of informed consent is soundly made by appeal to these two justifications. However, it is important to note that even if we concede this, the empirical evidence, suggesting that patients have problems when involved in the information giving and receiving elements of the informed consent process, still continues to exist. These problems are serious enough to raise the issue of whether it is actually possible to obtain informed consent in a real sense at all. Perhaps the conclusion will have to be that despite informed consent being a laudable aim, in reality it can at best only be partially achieved. Let us now consider some of the relevant empirical evidence.

4. Informed Consent: The Empirical Reality

We have seen that informed consent is popular amongst the public, that it can be morally justified through an appeal to autonomy and well-being, and that it has received growing ethical and legal support. However, there is good reason to be cautious about the role that informed consent has come to have in relation to healthcare, even if we think it is a good thing. This caution arises from the implications of the empirical evidence that can be gathered in relation to the effectiveness of attempts to gain informed consent in practice. In the rest of this section I will outline and discuss empirical evidence relating to a number of different aspects of informed consent.[17] However, before we do this I should, perhaps, enter a general caveat about empirical evidence and the way that it is used in ethical arguments. This qualification arises from the sense that we should always treat such evidence as provisional (as it can always be questioned or overturned in the future) and that we should note that different studies are of varying quality (as many are small scale and have various methodological limitations).[18] As a result of these factors, we should always be cautious in our arguments using empirical evidence, and we should take care not to over-generalize. However, we should also resist the temptation just to ignore empirical evidence related to an issue where it is available. It is too easy to suggest a course of ethical action and then just pay no attention to the fact that we have evidence that it is difficult or impossible to achieve that desired end. One important point to note about the empirical evidence in relation to informed consent is the scale of research on this issue. (For example, in a general review of the empirical studies published in relation to all areas of medical ethics, Jeremy Sugarman, R. Faden and J. Weinstein suggest that 16% of the total number of articles focused on informed consent, making this the most popular single topic.[19])

There are numerous examples of studies with implications for the pursuit of informed consent, and in this brief review I will only focus on evidence in three areas. The first relates to the way that pre-existing and background psychological factors and the experience of illness can influence decision-making. The second relates to evidence about general comprehension of significant pieces of information, and the third relates to evidence about understanding the relevant information through later recall.

A. Background and Influencing Factors

A key aspect of informed consent is that it is about communication between two different parties: physician and patient. In relation to this point, G. Kent reminds us that we should not ignore the fact that "social and psychological processes involved in communication between individuals need to be taken into account."[20] He argues that there is a need for anyone involved in obtaining informed consent to have knowledge of, and act upon, any relevant psychological evidence about problems in gaining the relevant patient understanding. He provides a good summary of many of the issues relating to how the psychological evidence bears upon the issue of informed consent. I will mention just two issues here.

The first is that psychologists have established that the way that information is provided to subjects influences their assessment of it. Examples might include the fact that people will tend to remember the first bit of evidence, or the riskiest, or that they might tend to be influenced in a particular direction by the way that the information is presented. Observation of such "framing effects" can be seen in a number of areas.[21] An example of clear relevance to this paper is the effect upon perceived risk of outcomes where the same risks are described in terms of survival rates or death rates.[22] Similar deformations upon the assessment of risk can be seen in studies that have noted the way that the probability of a negative outcome is given greater weight than its severity within judgment about risk.[23]

The second example is that it is now well recognized that the patient's pre-existing and background beliefs, attitudes, and values will influence the decisions that she makes. This means that such things as the patient's emotional state will make a difference to her decision. It often seems to be forgotten that patients are, generally, in the position that they are precisely because they are ill. Barrie R. Cassileth, R. V. Zupkis, K. Sutton-Smith, and V. March argue that understanding is at least partly related to the degree of illness of the patient: as the illness progresses patients understand less.[24] This seems completely plausible. Patients should not be assumed to be rational consumers with the ability to efficiently process a large amount of detailed and complex information and then make a decision based upon an objective determination of the best outcome for them. Although, of course, some will be able to do this, most will not. Tom Beauchamp and James Childress provide a plausible warning about ignoring this issue:

> Many patients cannot, in advance, adequately appreciate the nature of the pain, and many ill patients reach a point at which they can no longer balance with clear judgment the threat of pain against the benefits of surgery. At this point, they find the benefits of surgery overwhelmingly attractive, while devaluing the risks.[25]

In such a situation it is going to be difficult to give an informed consent however much information is forthcoming.

B. General Comprehension

There is also significant evidence that various factors mean that a patient's comprehension of the disclosed information is likely to be impeded. One example discussed by Kent is to do with evidence about the lack of "readability" of consent forms and information sheets.[26] Although in many cases these pieces of documentation will have been reviewed by lay people, there are a number of reasons why such countervailing factors can influence comprehension and recall of the information provided even when they are clearly written. For example Gert, Culver, and Clouser discuss a situation in which information is given to a patient in relation to a drug for a heart condition.[27] The patient is first told that it is commonly (85% of the time) associated with unpleasant side effects, but that it will reduce the chance of a heart attack by 50%. Many people might be tempted to run the risk of the harm when presented with such odds. However, the reduction in the possibility of heart attack has actually dropped from 1/200 to 1/100. Presented in this way it might look less rational to take the drug. Another example is provided by the work of H. J. Sutherland, G. A. Lockwood, D. L. Tritchler, F. Sem, L. Brooks, and J. E. Till,[28] that suggests that people seem to interpret key words routinely associated with discussion of risks and benefits (e.g. "usually," "frequently," "occasionally," and "rare") in very different ways. It is sometimes argued that evidence about risks can be translated into parallels with commonly experienced everyday events (for example, journey by car between two points, and so on) but this type of approach can also run into problems.[29]

C. Understanding and Recall of Information

Perhaps the most worrying message to come out of the research in this area is that a consistently large percentage of patients will later not be able to recall crucial information presented to them in either written or oral form as part of the informing process. For example, a study by E. M. Taylor, S. Parker, and S. P. Ramsay[30] looked at the understanding by patients of written information about a resuscitation policy in a New Zealand hospital. The study suggests that written information is not particularly helpful (at least within this type of context). Of the 401 patients interviewed, only 49% recalled being given the patient information booklet on admission and only 17% recalled reading the information about the resuscitation policy. Another example of such a study is that conducted by Cassileth and his colleagues.[31] This study focused on 200 cancer patients who filled in a questionnaire the day after they had opted for various forms of treatment. Only 60% appeared to understand the purpose and nature of the procedure, and only 55% were able to correctly state even one major risk or complication of the treatment option. Beauchamp and Childress also give a startling example of this problem when they quote from a study that suggested that over 50% of patients had forgotten that a particular procedure carried a high risk of death within a few weeks, although they were held to understand this just before the surgery.[32]

Of course, we should note that it is not clear that understanding of the relevant facts in relation to a consent are tested most effectively by investigating the recipient's recall of what was said or read at some earlier time. However, the best of this literature tests comprehension in these terms very soon after the moment of consenting, and in the absence of any other methodological tools it is the best we have. Wear summarizes the literature on this issue as follows:

> [The] low levels of recall, and the absence of any study showing high recall of even the "essentials," question any optimistic view of informed consent.[33]

At the very least the supporter of informed consent should be concerned that so many participants in informed consent interactions are unable to recall salient details even after short periods.

5. What Should We Do Now?

The response often given to this type of evidence is that we just need to give more information as part of the process of obtaining an informed consent—as though the issue were just one of poor communication. On this view we can be more aware of the different problems and take them into account in practice. In some cases this might be true. However, in other cases it looks as though a more serious remedy is required, for two reasons. The first is that the very number of different problems suggests that it will prove difficult to respond to all of the issues and, secondly, many of the concerns arise from the way that the information is processed rather than the fact that there is a lack of information as such. The message of the published evidence seems to be that we need to consider more radical solutions.

One possibility, in the spirit of informed consent, might be to try to use a more individual-oriented approach such as that provided by decision analysis. For example, P. Ubel and George Loewenstein[34] recognize that whilst the model of informed consent is one that allows the individual patient to be the one to choose which medical option fits with her own values, the problem is that in many situations the range of options (each with its own risks of harm and potential benefits) to be absorbed means that there is too much information for the individual to meaningfully process and use as the basis for a decision. This view is supported by empirical psychological evidence and suggests that even when an individual is clear about what her priorities are in terms of her values (and this is a big assumption), she is still likely to find it difficult to choose which medical option is the best fit for those values. Ubel and Loewenstein give the example of choosing between four different cancer screening tests (flexible sigmoidoscopy, colonoscopy, barium enema, and fecal occult blood testing). They argue that if

> the information physicians give patients does not help patients make choices that fit their values, then informed consent doctrine loses much of its moral justification. To meet the moral goals of informed consent, physicians need to find a method to combine patients' values with medical facts in a way that produces superior medical decisions.[35]

Their paper is a discussion of the possible benefits of using formal decision-making tools (such as decision analysis) as an aid to patients faced with the need to decide which medical option is most appropriate in terms of their values. It also usefully discusses some so-called "intuitive" factors (such as regret, fear, and hope), which, it is argued, should be incorporated into decision analysis. Decision analysis might well be useful for an individual attempting to weigh different options before arriving at a decision about which one is best. However, given the complexity of this approach, it can hardly provide a solution to the problem of poor understanding of the information relevant to healthcare decision making.

The empirical evidence in relation to informed consent has had no discernible impact on the way that bioethicists and policy makers have approached the issue of informed consent. The consensus view is still that we should insist upon it. This seems odd given the consistency of the message emerging from the published empirical studies. It might be that modifications can be introduced into the process of gaining informed consent so that all the possible problems can be overcome. If this is the case, it would seem reasonable to assume that the supporters of informed consent would address the issues raised to ensure the best possible chance of the desired outcome. After all, if it is the case that informed consent is morally required, then surely we have an obligation to try as hard as we can to achieve it. There seems to be little evidence of this having occurred, and it is not enough simply to suggest that doctors undertake more training in communication skills. Even if there were evidence of the empirical studies being taken seriously and addressed in practice, problems in gaining truly informed consent are likely to remain. This is because of the deep-rooted psychological nature of some of the issues uncovered by the empirical research.

Another option is to carry on with the present policy of acting as though we are getting true informed consent. Such an approach might be defensible if we have evidence that people want us to do this, and it in turn does no harm. However, an alternative response would be to argue that this view is unethical because we are pretending to do something when we know that in a large percentage of cases it is difficult if not impossible to achieve the desired end. On such a view, it is offensive to persist with such pretence, and the conclusion must be that we should give up trying to do the impossible.

6. Conclusion

Informed consent is an issue with a high profile. It has had a prominent position in the bioethics literature of the last thirty years, and has come to be seen as essential in both a clinical and a research context by public bodies such as the National Health Service in the United Kingdom. Despite this high profile, it is important to acknowledge and take seriously the empirical research of relevance to this issue. Even such a supporter of the idea of informed consent as Wear is forced to conclude that while various positive effects such as "enhanced compliance, coping, and a diminished experience of anxiety and anticipated pain, seem to clearly derive from informed consent," the overall aim of producing the "informed patient as decision maker has just not materialized."[36]

It is clear from the review of the evidence above that more research needs to be conducted to explore the potential problems with the understanding of information given as part of the process of obtaining an informed consent. In the light of the evidence, as things stand at the moment, we have good grounds for thinking that it does not make sense to put so much weight on gaining an informed consent. While it might be the case that informed consent can survive as a requirement, it might have to be radically revised as a practice. We must certainly accept the limitations of the concept, and at the very least explore ways to improve the process. The present almost universal insistence upon giving an informed consent in clinical and research contexts does not seem appropriate given the evidence of the clash of this bioethical ideal with empirical reality.

NOTES

1. *Informed Consent in Medical Research*, ed. Len Doyal and Jeffrey Tobias (London: BMJ Books, 2001), pp. 3–4.
2. www.wma.net/e/
3. www.doh.gov.uk/consent
4. www.bma.org.uk/ap.nsf/Content/consenttk2
5. www.gmc-uk.org/standards/default.htm
6. Tom Beauchamp and James Childress, *Principles of Biomedical Ethics* (Oxford: Oxford University Press, 5th ed., 2001), pp. 79–80.

7. Bernard Gert, Charles M. Culver, and K. Danner Clouser, *Bioethics: A Return to Fundamentals* (Oxford: Oxford University Press, 1997), p. 151.

8. Stephen Wear, *Informed Consent: Patient Autonomy and Clinical Beneficence* (Washington, DC: Georgetown University Press, 2nd ed., 1998).

9. Allen E. Buchanan and Dan W. Brock, *Deciding For Others: The Ethics of Surrogate Decision Making* (Cambridge: Cambridge University Press, 1989).

10. Mark R. Wicclair, "Patient Decision-Making Capacity and Risk," *Bioethics*, 5:2 (1991), pp. 91–104; Dan W. Brock, "Decision-Making Competence and Risk," *Bioethics*, 5:2 (1991), pp. 105–112; Becky Cox White, *Competence to Consent* (Washington, DC: Georgetown University Press, 1994); G. Cale, "Risk-Related Standards of Competence: Continuing the Debate Over the Risk-Related Standards of Competence," *Bioethics*, 13:2 (1999), pp. 131–148; Mark R. Wicclair, "The Continuing Debate Over Risk-Related Standards of Competence," *Bioethics*, 13: 2 (1999), pp. 149–153.; Tom Buller, "Competency and Risk-Relativity," *Bioethics*, 15:2 (2001), pp. 93–109.

11. Lord Chancellor's Department, *Making Decisions: The Government's Proposals for Making Decisions on Behalf of Mentally Incapacitated Adults* (London: The Stationery Office, 1999); Angus Dawson, "Advance Directives," *General Practice and Ethics: Uncertainty and Responsibility*, ed. Christopher Dowrick and Lucy Frith (London: Routledge, 1999).

12. Dan W. Brock, "Informed Consent," *Health Care Ethics: An Introduction*, ed. Donald van de Veer and Tom Regan (Philadelphia: Temple University Press, 1987), pp. 98–126.

13. John Stuart Mill, *On Liberty* (Mineola, NY: Dover Publications, 2002).

14. *Paternalism*, ed. Rolf Sartorius (Minneapolis: University of Minnesota Press, 1983).

15. R. J. Alfidi, "Informed Consent: A Study of Patient Reaction," *Journal of the American Medical Association*, 216:8 (1971), pp.1325–1329; W. M. Strull, B. Lo, and G. Charles, "Do Patients Want to Participate in Medical Decision-Making?," *Journal of the American Medical Association*, 252:21 (1984), pp. 2990–2994.

16. *Informed Consent*, ed. Doyal and Tobias; President's Advisory Committee, *The Human Radiation Experiments* (Oxford: Oxford University Press, 1996).

17. Jeremy Sugarman, D. McCrory, D. Powell, A. Krasny, E. Ball, and C. Cassell, "Empirical Research on Informed Consent," *Hastings Center Report*, 29:1 Supplement, S1-S42 (1999).

18. Jeremy Sugarman, R. Faden, and J. Weinstein, "A Decade of Empirical Research in Medical Ethics," *Methods in Medical Ethics*, ed. Jeremy Sugarman and Daniel P. Sulmasy (Washington, DC: Georgetown University Press, 2001), pp. 19–30; Wear, *Informed Consent*, chapter 3.

19. Sugarman *et al*, "A Decade of Empirical Research in Medical Ethics," p. 23.

20. Gerry Kent, (1996) "Shared Understandings for Informed Consent: The Relevance of Psychological Research on the Provision of Information," *Social Science and Medicine*, 43:10 (1996), p.1518.

21. A. Tversky and D. Kahneman, "The Framing of Decisions and the Psychology of Choice," *Science*, 211:4481 (1981), pp. 453–458; A. Tversky and D.

Kahneman, "Choices, Values, and Frames," *American Psychologist*, 39:4 (1984), pp. 341–50.

22. B. J. McNeil, S. G. Pauker, H. C. Sox, and A. Tversky (1982) "On the Elicitation of Preferences for Alternative Therapies," *New England Journal of Medicine*, 306:21 (1982), pp. 1259–1262.

23. K. Hopper, P. Houts, M. McCauslin, Y. Matthews, and R. Sefczek, "Patients' Attitudes Towards Informed Consent for Intravenous Contrast-Media," *Investigative Radiology*, 27:5 (1992), pp. 362–366; J. F. Merz, M. J. Druzdzel, and D. J. Mazur, "Verbal Expressions of Probability in Informed Consent Litigation," *Medical Decision Making*, 11:4 (1991), pp. 273–281.

24. B. R. Cassileth, R. V. Zupkis, K. Sutton-Smith, and V. March, "Informed Consent: Why are Its Goals Imperfectly Realized?," *New England Journal of Medicine*, 302:16 (1980), pp. 896–900.

25. Beauchamp and Childress, *Principles of Biomedical Ethics*, p. 89.

26. Kent, "Shared Understandings for Informed Consent," p.1518.

27. Gert *et al.*, *Bioethics*, p.165.

28. H. J. Sutherland, G. A. Lockwood, D. L. Tritchler, F. Sem, L. Brooks, and J. Till, "Communicating Probabilistic Information to Cancer Patients: Is there 'Noise' on the Line?," *Social Science and Medicine*, 32:6 (1991), pp. 725–731.

29. S. Lichtenstein, P. Slovic, B. Fischoff, M. Layman, and B. Combs, "Judging Frequency of Lethal Events," *Journal of Experimental Psychology*, 4 (1978), pp. 55–78.

30. E. M. Taylor, S. Parker, and M. P. Ramsay, "Patients' Receipt and Understanding of Written Information About a Resuscitation Policy," *Bioethics*, 12:1 (1998), pp. 64–76.

31. Cassileth *et al.*, "Informed Consent."

32. Beauchamp and Childress, *Principles of Biomedical Ethics*, p. 90, p. 110.

33. Wear, *Informed Consent*, p. 53

34. P. Ubel and G. Loewenstein, "The Role of Decision Analysis in Informed Consent: Choosing between Intuition and Systematicity," *Social Science and Medicine*, 44:5 (1997), pp. 647–656.

35. *Ibid.*, p. 648.

36. Wear, *Informed Consent*, p. 55.

Nine

WHAT EMPIRICAL BIOETHICS CAN LEARN FROM EMPIRICAL BUSINESS ETHICS

Søren Holm

1. Introduction

Bioethics and business ethics are related fields. They can both be described as applied ethics, and are both concerned with ethical problems that occur within a set of socially important practices (healthcare and business respectively). They both attempt to make claims that are supposed to be relevant for practitioners in the fields of interest, and they both build on the same standard set of ethical theories developed in moral philosophy, or in the early days of applied philosophy (the principlist approach is, for instance popular in both fields). In both fields there has also over the years been an increase in the number of empirical studies performed. The empirical trend in business ethics is older than the empirical trend in bioethics. This can probably be explained by the different environments in which the two disciplines developed, and the concomitant differences in views about academic merit ("pure philosophy" not being highly rated in business schools). In business ethics, the proportion of empirical work appears to have stabilized at around 30–40% of the papers published in the main journal, the *Journal of Business Ethics*,[1] whereas in bioethics it is still increasing.

This chapter builds on an analysis of the empirical studies in the two fields with regard to:

- The questions asked.
- The theoretical frameworks.
- The methodology.
- The actual conduct of the study.
- The conclusions drawn.

It is uncontroversial that many of our ethical arguments rely on empirical premises of different kinds. We often need to know something about the world in which the moral agent is supposed to act, something about the general characteristics of moral agents, something about the limitations for action imposed by nature, culture or institutions, and something about how we can effectively influence decision-making and action. This is true both for the basic ethical analysis, and when we move on to suggest changes in legislation or institutional arrangements.

Traditionally these empirical premises have been imported from other fields of study like sociology, anthropology, or psychology. The current trend towards more empirical studies within the different fields of applied ethics can probably be explained in several ways. One explanation is the broadening of the disciplinary background of people working in the field. Another is that as the ethical questions considered become more specific, it becomes more difficult to find answers to the empirical questions in other disciplines. Some of the empirical premises needed for an analysis of whether euthanasia should be legalized may never have been interesting enough outside the context of this specific ethical question to become subjects of study by sociologists, and so on.

But if empirical studies are to be valuable contributions to the field, they have to ask relevant questions, use suitable methodologies, and be well conducted. They also ideally have to build on, or at least relate to, earlier studies, so that over time a coherent body of work is developed.

2. Bioethics and Business Ethics—the Main Differences

Since this chapter is written for a readership presumably cognizant of the state of bioethics, I will here focus on empirical business ethics. The main difference between empirical bioethics and empirical business ethics is that, whereas empirical bioethics is almost exclusively exploratory and descriptive in nature, in empirical business ethics it is possible to find many more studies that are either experimental or have some clearly stated theory-backed hypothesis that is being investigated. This is by no means to say that this type of research is dominant in business ethics, but just that it is more common than in bioethics.

A full survey of the methodology of both fields would almost certainly be as depressing as the systematic analysis published by D. M. Randall and A. M. Gibson in 1990 of the methodology of ninety-four empirical business ethics studies published from 1961 to 1989.[2] They found consistent severe weaknesses in almost all of the areas of methodology they evaluated, apart from choice of study population and data analysis. A main weakness in the business ethics literature is that many studies use students as their research population because these are easily available and can be induced or coerced to answer, ensuring large samples and high response rates. This is clearly problematic, since students lack the experience of "real businessmen." Here empirical bioethics appears to be in a better position, with a large proportion of studies actually studying the practitioners at the coalface.

This methodological criticism does not entail that there are no good papers to be found if we look carefully. What can be found in reasonably large numbers in the business ethics literature are studies that not only investigate what relevant people think, believe, feel, or do, but which also try to link this with some meaningful background variables—variables that are more likely to contribute to our understanding of why people make different decisions or perform different actions than those of age, sex, or stated religion. In a recent review of (English language) studies assessing ethical decision-making in business, T. W. Loe and co-workers are for instance able to find fifteen studies investigating the relationship between ethical awareness and ethical decision-making, twenty-one studies looking at the influence of a person's moral philosophical orientation on decision-making (an interesting finding here appears to be that only persons able to use both deontological and consequentialist approaches are able satisfactorily to resolve all types of business ethical problems; satisfaction with resolution of problems here is measured by the respondents' self-evaluation), seventeen studies studying the effect of Codes of Ethics, fifteen studying the effect of rewards and sanctions, and eighteen looking at the influence of organizational culture and climate.[3] It would be impossible to identify any similar reasonably coherent body of work in bioethics.

Another important field of study in business ethics, which lacks a parallel in bioethics, is large-scale studies of the often negative effects of ethically questionable practices. There is, for instance, a thriving research program looking at how corruption in general, and the institutionalization of bribery in particular, have negative macro-economic effects in those countries where corruption is widespread. The results of this research show that corruption in business is not only immoral, but that it also can be "proven" to be economically counterproductive at the societal level. It is simply not the case that corruption is the grease that lets the economy run smoothly. The research shows that it is more like the sand that stops the machine from working.

Similar work is lacking in bioethics with regard to the most common ethically problematic behaviors in healthcare practice. This lacuna allows people to continue to put forward arguments along the lines of "Yes, it might be ethically bad, but it is still pragmatically useful."

3. Some Concrete Illustrations

Let me further illustrate the strengths and weaknesses of empirical studies in business ethics with two recent studies. Most of us tend to believe that if people are more ethically aware they will also make better decisions, and eventually perform better acts (or if we do not believe it deep down, we are at least prone to say things like that when we try to "sell" ethics and philosophy of medicine teaching.) But this is clearly an empirically testable hypothesis, although it needs some specification before it can be tested.

A Norwegian study published in 2001 tests two hypotheses derived from this main hypothesis.[4] It tests whether strong moral attitudes negatively affect moral reasoning, and whether good moral reasoning differentially influences policy-decisions and action-decisions. Both hypotheses were, to the surprise of the researcher, rejected, and it was found that the main effect of moral reasoning on decision-making was that persons with good moral reasoning showed far greater variation in decision-making than persons with low moral reasoning scores. The author reasonably concluded that either our measurement instruments for the constructs involved are wrong, or we need to think again about the relationship between moral reasoning and action.

A study from the United States published in 2000 examined the interrelationship between ethical sensitivity and moral reasoning or development. Most models for ethical decision-making have the recognition and identification of an ethical problem as their first step, and cognitive processing of the identified problem as their second step. It is therefore important to investigate whether these two constructs are separate or whether they are connected. Most writers assume that they are connected and that persons with better sensitivity also display better reasoning. In order to study this, the researchers studied the direct relationship between sensitivity and reasoning, but also the relationship of each of the constructs with a range of five other constructs: relativism, empathy, deontological orientation, teleological orientation, and Machiavellianism. A hypothesis was put forward concerning the direction of each of these relationships. In the study it was found that whereas all hypotheses concerning ethical reasoning were corroborated by the findings, none of the hypotheses concerning ethical sensitivity was corroborated, and the authors are forced to conclude that ethical sensitivity, along with the empirical evidence, "continues to suggest that no relationship between the constructs exists in spite of the strong intuitive appeal to an association between them."[5]

What these two studies share is primarily a commitment to a theory- or hypothesis-driven research process, and a willingness to build on and extend work already done in the field. Let us imagine that someone in a few years is going to write a new review of empirical studies assessing ethical decision-making in business. Because the two studies we have just looked at are theory-based, such a review can not only mention their specific results, but can also discuss these results in relation to other studies based on the same theories.

These studies are far from perfect. In both cases we may well query the instruments used to measure the central constructs. Both for instance use versions of James Rest's DIT-test to measure development in moral reasoning,[6] and this test is for many tainted by belonging to the Kohlberg tradition of cognitive moral development theory. But both studies could have been conducted with a utilitarian, virtue theoretical, or communitarian test for moral reasoning instead (or perhaps a mega-instrument incorporating all the different constructs of moral reasoning).

4. Conclusion

The main lesson of this analysis is that empirical bioethics can learn from emp-irical business ethics that description is not enough. We have to move beyond studies simply reporting that x% of physicians in country y think that euthanasia should be legalized, to studies investigating what their reasons are, and whether these reasons can be connected to more overarching moral constructs. Is there a difference between people with a deontological and a consequentialist orientation? Is there a difference between those who have participated in ethics courses and those who have not? Is there a difference between paternalists and non-paternalists?

We also need to be more careful in planning our studies in such a way that they can be compared with studies of the same topic performed by other researchers. Although important insight and knowledge can be produced by the single, excellent research project, there are in most cases significant gains to be found in the accumulation of knowledge which occurs if current research builds on prior research, and does not try to reinvent the methodological wheel in every new project.

NOTES

1. Denis Collins, "The Quest to Improve the Human Condition: The First 1500 Articles Published in *Journal of Business Ethics*," *Journal of Business Ethics*, 26:1 (July 2000), pp. 1–73.

2. Donna M. Randall and Annetta M. Gibson, "Methodology in Business Ethics Research: A Review and Critical Assessment," *Journal of Business Ethics*, 9:6 (June 1990), pp. 457–471.

3. Terry W. Loe, Linda Ferrell, and Phylis Mansfield, "A Review of Empirical Studies Assessing Ethical Decision Making in Business," *Journal of Business Ethics*, 25:3 (June 2000), pp. 185–204.

4. Einar Marnburg, "The Questionable Use of Moral Development Theory in Studies of Business Ethics: Discussion and Empirical Findings," *Journal of Business Ethics*, 32:4 (August 2001), pp. 275–283.

5. John R. Sparks and J. P. Merenski, "Recognition-Based Measures of Ethical Sensitivity and Reformulated Cognitive Moral Development: An Examination and Evidence of Nomological Validity," *Teaching Business Ethics* 4:4 (Winter 2000), pp. 359–377.

6. *Moral Development: Advances in Research and Theory*, ed. James Rest (New York, NY: Praeger, 1986).

Ten

ON CORPORATE ETHICAL RESPONSIBILITY, STAKEHOLDER VALUE, AND STRICT LIABILITY IN BIOTECHNOLOGY

Jukka Kilpi

1. Business Ethics

The ethical responsibility of the corporation consists of more than a mere duty to obey the law. Ethical responsibility is founded on values that fall within the spheres of morals and ethics. Normative ethics, or moral philosophy, analyses values, defines general principles on which values are based, and applies rational arguments to point out which values are right or good.

Applied ethics, as the name of the discipline suggests, is the area of normative ethics that explores conflicts of values in specific domains of human action. Medical ethics and bioethics are examples of established and well-known domains of applied ethics. Business ethics is also a well-established area of applied ethics. Since the 1980s it has been a vital ingredient of the academic curriculum and research, initially in the United States of America and more recently in Europe. Lately, business ethics has also become a more common item on the agenda of large corporations. In particular, multinational corporations include ethical steering and control processes as integral parts of their quality and management systems. Simultaneously, regulators are drafting legislation that will make ethical auditing obligatory for public companies in the same way as environmental auditing has already been introduced to company reports.

In spite of this development it is still common for "business ethics" to be regarded as an oxymoron. How can business have anything to do with ethics? Business is about making money, and must somehow be morally suspicious, must it not? This pessimistic view is surprisingly often taken, even by those whose life and career concentrates on doing honest business.

To see business and morals as alien, or even opposite, to each other is a serious and unfortunate aberration—but one with a very long history. Aristotle, for instance, considered money-making associated with trade as dirty activity, as his discussion in Book I of *The Politics* shows:

> Money-making then, as we have said, is of two kinds; one which is necessary and acceptable, which we may call administrative; the other, the commercial, which depends on exchange, is justly regarded with

> disapproval, since it arises not from nature but from men's dealings with each other.[1]

This Aristotelian fallacy is still very much alive among philosophers and has boosted a school of business ethics called virtue ethics.

The mission of virtue ethicists is to introduce altruistic values into business in order to counter-balance the egoistic greed intrinsically dominating that activity. Virtue ethics emphasizes, in the spirit of Aristotle, that the essence of human nature is altruistic promotion of other people's good and, therefore, altruism also has to be the final goal of business. This means that corporate ethical responsibility should dampen economic doctrines based on profit, competition, and the promotion of individual interests.

However, if we employ the tools of academic philosophy in the research of business practices and values, the hollowness of Aristotelian virtue ethics' taking business as immoral or amoral is soon revealed. The systematic analysis of values and their conflicts in business should start with a look at the major traditions of philosophical ethics. They relate to issues on three different levels.

2. Fundamental Issues of Philosophical Ethics

Three different levels of fundamental philosophical issues are usually identified in ethics:

- *Metaethics*: Can we rank values by means of argument and analysis? Are values truth-apt or not?
- *Normative ethics*: What values and moral principles are the good and right ones and what establishes their goodness or rightness?
- *Applied ethics*: Values and principles applied to practical life.

In philosophical research and argumentation these three levels are interconnected. An answer to the metaethical issues has an impact on the results of the normative account, and so also to the practical implementation of values. From the point of view of a philosophical theory, then, metaethics is not irrelevant when a view of the ethical responsibility of the corporation is formulated. This suggests that we should start the analysis of corporate ethical responsibility by summing up the answers major traditions of moral philosophy give to the fundamental metaethical problem of the truth-aptness of values.

The oldest defense of the objectivity of values is the claim that values do objectively exist in an ontological sense. Hence the name "natural law" or "natural rights philosophy": values exist in the world as independent entities, like trees, or animals, or human beings. Two examples of alternative ways in which these independent entities have been claimed to exist are Plato's immutable ideas and Thomas Aquinas's doctrine of God's will.

Mainstream philosophy and jurisprudence rejected natural law and natural rights centuries ago.[2] The criticism points out that, unlike with other objects of nature, it is impossible to have direct perceptions of values. Perceiving them immediately is possible only with the aid of strong belief, and belief is not sufficient for an argument supporting a rational theory. In the absence of empirical evidence for independently existing objective values, natural law or natural rights do not carry enough moral weight to establish corporate ethical responsibility.

Utilitarianism, initiated by David Hume, was the British empiricists' reply to natural law philosophy. Utilitarianism takes the maximization of the satisfaction of interests as the key to rightness and goodness. It is a clear and convincing moral theory that still exercises a strong influence in philosophy. The most serious criticism against utilitarianism is that the theory may be used to justify otherwise unfounded harm imposed upon one person, if this increases the happiness of the many. In other words, utilitarianism may yield support to actions that we see as offending some persons' rights. It is an inadequate theory, as it is incapable of giving an individual's rights the status we actually do give them in our intuitions and everyday moral judgments.

An alternative to utilitarianism is deontological ethics, or the ethics of duty. Its centerpiece is the intrinsic value of rights and duties, and respect for moral principles promulgating them. Immanuel Kant is often cited as the most prominent deontological ethicist. He called the highest moral principle the "categorical imperative." Its contents echo the ancient golden rule of morals: always treat a person as you would wish other persons to treat you in a similar situation.

Kant derived his theory from his account of human beings as autonomous and rational beings. Our autonomy and rationality are the foundation that makes us capable of respecting moral principles, and they are also the foundation of the objectivity of values. Even so, values do not have any objective existence outside the realm of human reason. Kant stood against natural law philosophers, while at the same time defending metaethical objectivism.

From the point of view of modern ethics, subjectivism has a close relation to twentieth century empiricism, and its offspring analytic philosophy. The most distinguished Finnish philosopher of all time, G. H. von Wright, gained his reputation from research purporting to dispute the claim that values are truth-apt.[3] According to von Wright and his analytic colleagues, values are conventions and practices grown out of social patterns of life. They can be analyzed and the inherent logic of value hierarchies can be assessed but, ultimately, disputes over the rightness or truth of values are irresolvable.

Analytic philosophy promoted normative ethical research in setting the standards of systematic, logical, and lucid analysis. This is evident in the manner that these standards are still employed in Anglo-American normative ethics to formulate arguments seeking to show moral principles to be true or right. Also, more recent analytic philosophy has established ways to allow for the truth-aptness of values.[4]

In addition to these positive impacts, analytic philosophy succeeded in blurring the field of normative philosophy. Some philosophers, who have adopted the basically subjectivist metaethical idea of analytic philosophy, have felt that participation in the normative debate is their prime responsibility. Since they do not think that rational knowledge of values can be attained, they have thrown themselves into normative discourse by propounding their subjective opinions and preferences. The values they have stood for have sometimes been backed less by normative arguments and analysis than by their personal credentials as philosophers gained in areas outside normative ethics.

The result has been that the subjectivism associated with early analytical philosophy has infused normative debate on moral principles with vagueness and irrationality. This applies to business ethics as well. Virtue ethics, already mentioned above, is a good example: business is requested to adopt virtues without a proper analysis of what business is about and without a rational justification of the virtues glorified.

Another major problem with virtue ethics is its inherent lack of challenge: if the criterion of a virtue and, consequently, the criterion of an ethically responsible corporation, is that it altruistically promotes the welfare of other persons, the solution is too simple and single-minded. As virtue ethics does not offer rational arguments for altruistic ethical responsibility, a person who does not share the virtuous Aristotelian view of altruistic human essence is not given any reason to adopt altruism and act accordingly.

It has been common to accommodate Aristotle in the objectivist metaethical camp, and quite rightly so, as his teleological ethics puts the emphasis on human nature and its perfection in virtuous life. However, I have included him among the subjectivists because of the epistemic and methodological character of his account of human nature and virtues. He relies too much on moral insight instead of argument, and substitutes moral psychology for moral theory in stating his views.[5] The consequence is that the truth or goodness of the virtues he stipulates as the prerequisite of human perfection and moral goodness are founded on his authority and insight, instead of on argument and analysis. Although a metaethical objectivist in an ontological sense, Aristotle is an epistemological and methodological subjectivist in the way that he establishes ethically valuable norms.

This basically subjectivist method is carried on by contemporary virtue ethicists who take Aristotle as their ultimate authority, granting them a license to beg the question for virtues they advocate. This is a pity because, as Jonathan Jacobs has recently noted, virtue-centered teleological considerations could well be included in ethical discourse without potentially embarrassing Aristotelian grand insights:

> Now it would appear that we can retain the teleology of this and that project, or concern, or aspiration, but the metaphysical essentialist quality of teleology is unbelievable. This is one crucial way in which moral theory has taken over and subordinated or domesticated virtue. We can talk of virtues as dispositions to act for moral reasons but not as actualizations of objective excellences.[6]

3. Toward a Rational Normative Discourse on Corporate Ethical Responsibility

What makes normative ethics challenging is the provision of rational arguments that systematically purport to show why those who disagree should change their thinking and values. The arguments even have to show why sometimes it is right to use compulsion, for instance by means of laws, to force those who disagree on a principle nevertheless to live by that principle. Applied to corporate ethical responsibility this means that we have to provide arguments which show that the corporation, and those persons who act on its behalf, have to bear ethical responsibility even when they, quite legitimately, are motivated by profit and the satisfaction of their interests.

Economics and anthropology take humans as rational individuals who endeavor to satisfy their interests.[7] This does not exclude the human ability to pay respect to moral principles or choose an altruistic course of action, but it is reasonable to build moral and ethical responsibility on a concept of human nature that matches, as this one does, the paradigms of science. A normative theory is seriously weakened as rational philosophy if it adopts some other idea of human nature. It is also more likely that a normative theory that rests on an unrealistic view of mankind will face insurmountable difficulties when put into practice.

In this spirit, a quick evaluation of the major traditions of philosophical ethics suggests that the most promising theories for the analysis of corporate ethical responsibility are utilitarianism and deontological ethics. The utilitarian fundamentals are straightforward and practical: the corporation has to bear ethical responsibility if its consequences are useful, and the measure of usefulness may be, for instance, happiness, pleasure, or satisfaction of interests.

Utilitarianism is a strong basis for corporate ethical responsibility, but it is not a comprehensive theory. For instance, it leaves open the question as to what economic or distributive system is best—although the benefits of competitive markets are hard to ignore when the satisfaction of interests is assessed. It can be concluded, however, that a utilitarian would never make the maximization of profits the only issue for which the corporation should be ethically responsible. Corporate actions have an impact on a large number of persons, and corporations must bear the responsibility of the consequences of their actions in regard to all these affected stakeholders.

The core problem of utilitarianism as a philosophical theory is that it sometimes justifies the violation of the rights of some individuals in order to achieve the satisfaction of some other individuals' interests. This sets utilitarianism into conflict with deontological ethics, the cornerstone of which is rights founded on personal autonomy and rationality. Rights generate corporate ethical responsibility in the deontological sense too: on the one hand, autonomous persons have the right to freedom, including freedom to do business, whilst on the other hand they should carry out this freedom only through actions that respect the rights of others. In the corporate world, this translates into an ethical responsibility not to violate the rights of other agents.

In conclusion, ethics offers rival theories about the basis of corporate moral responsibility. Fundamentally, these rival theories propound different views of the human being as a moral agent. Utilitarianism and deontological ethics put the emphasis on the individual and his or her interests or rights, while virtue ethics focuses on social bonds and altruistic motives and ends. In order better to assess corporate ethical responsibility we should, next, go deeper into the concept of moral agency, and examine what kind of agent the corporation is in the web of interests, rights, and ends.

4. Shareholder Value versus Stakeholder Value

The ability to act intentionally is a necessary condition of an agent's attaining an ethically sensible status of moral agency. In other words, if an agent is not capable of intentions and of guiding her actions according to her will, she cannot influence her course of action, and cannot be held morally responsible for it either. The other side of the coin is that an agent capable of intentions is a moral person who bears responsibility for her actions. So, the question whether the corporation is ethically responsible reverts to the question of whether the corporation is a person.

Nobel prize winning economist Milton Friedman denied corporate personhood some decades ago in his classic article, "The Social Responsibility of Business is to Increase its Profits."[8] Friedman's core claim is that profit maximization exhausts the social responsibility of business. He sees the corporation as an aggregate of the individuals who own it. It can have no moral responsibility, except maybe a general duty to obey the law, apart from the purpose for which it has been set up, that purpose usually being the making of profit. The corporation is not a person and so cannot bear any general ethical responsibility.

Friedman's view has been the target of strong criticism. American philosopher Peter French has advocated a completely opposite view to Friedman: that the corporation is a full-fledged moral person.[9] French argues that corporate actions are irreducible to the actions of individuals, and that corporations do have an inbuilt decision-making structure that is capable of intentions and intentional actions. The corporation is more than a mere aggregate of individuals, it is a moral person and a moral agent.

French's argument has received wide recognition, but it has also been subjected to crushing criticism. French builds his theory on the linguistic fact that we ascribe intentions, and therefore personhood, to corporations in our language. This to French, in a Davidsonian vein, is enough to establish the existence of a corporate mind independent of any individual persons' minds. French's critics focus on this and claim that we may ascribe properties to entities without assuming that the ascribed properties exist in those entities in any ontological sense. Therefore, linguistic projections do not create moral persons or moral agents.

Thomas Donaldson, Kenneth Goodpaster, and Patricia Werhane[10] are renowned American business ethicists who have developed alternative theories that recognize our ascriptions of responsibility and intentions to corporations; establish corporate agency and social responsibility; but fall short of granting the corporation a fully independent personhood. According to these philosophers, it is rational to project ethical responsibility onto corporations, as not all corporate actions are reducible to actions of individuals. However, these projections do not make corporations independent persons, but give them what Patricia Werhane calls secondary autonomy and personhood, which is sufficient to make corporations ethically responsible for their actions. Therefore, in addition to shareholders' interest, a corporation has to pay respect to the interests of all of its stakeholders. This line of thought is now known as *stakeholder value* philosophy, and it has gained considerable ground in ethics, business, and politics, at the expense of the Friedmanite shareholder value approach.

5. The Corporation as a Nexus of Contracts: Responsibility toward the Members of the Network

So it is a widely held view in contemporary business ethics that the corporation is not an independent moral person but, even so, is ethically responsible for the promotion of its stakeholders' interests and welfare. The concept of "stakeholder" is taken to cover everybody associated, one way or another, with the corporate web. What is the nature of this broad ethical stakeholder responsibility? Is it related to altruism, like virtue ethics suggests, or can it be justified without giving up the idea of human beings as rational individuals who strive to satisfy their own interests? Much of the hottest debate in contemporary business ethics revolves around this question.

It is reasonable to argue that the answer should be based on a notion of the corporation that is accepted in science. Granted this, we should not reject the view of self-interested human rationality because, as noted above, it is the paradigm of economics and anthropology. It is desirable to stick with the self-interested view of human nature, because discrepancy with empirical science would weaken an ethical theory.

In applying the paradigm of self-interested rationality to the corporation, we should note that forty years ago when Milton Friedman first published his classic paper making shareholder interests the centerpiece of business ethics, economics and jurisprudence took the corporation to be an aggregate of self-interested individuals. However, more recently both economics[11] and jurisprudence[12] have proceeded towards the theory of the corporation as a nexus of contracts. If we, accordingly, start the assessment of the ethical responsibility of the corporation from its fundamental nature as a contractual network, it looks more obvious that the interests of all the parties of the web are ethically meaningful. Among these parties are shareholders, employees, management, directors, customers, suppliers, local authorities, state, and financiers, to mention just a few of the more obvious examples. We are led to the conclusion that stakeholder value philosophy is not only widely supported in contemporary normative research but is compatible with modern science's paradigm as to human and corporate character. This compatibility—or "open architecture" to use modern Information Technology business jargon—is a good indication that the corporation is ethically responsible not only to its shareholders for its actions, but to all its stakeholders.

6. Promise as the Foundation of a Contract

Why does the corporation's responsibility to all its stakeholders have an ethical flavor? Since we are dealing with contracts, would judicial responsibility not be sufficient? These questions may be tackled with help from jurisprudence, which widely accepts the view that contracts are based on promises.[13] This makes ethics unavoidable. Promising is an action infused with ethics: promises carry a moral obligation to keep the promise.

Next, then, we may ask upon what the morally binding character of promises is based? The answers given to this question vary depending on their association with one or another major tradition of moral philosophy. The most interesting theories of promising are the utilitarian ones emphasizing the usefulness of promise-keeping, deontological ethics connecting promises to the autonomous will and moral agency of a person, and contractual thinking explaining promises as conventions of social interaction. Without examining these theories in any further detail we may conclude that none of the theories challenges, *prima facie*, the moral principle that promises should be kept. This unanimity, not so frequent in philosophy, is a good reason to accept that contracts, as a species of promises, contain moral obligations. Therefore, the corporation, which by its very nature is a nexus of contracts, has an ethical responsibility to take into account all the interests that come under the impact of corporate actions through the contractual network that constitutes the acting corporate agent. The corporation is ethically responsible to all its stakeholders.

7. Stakeholder Value and Strict Liability in Biotechnology

What are the bioethical implications of the corporation's stakeholder responsibility? In this chapter I hope to point out some of them in regard to genetic modification (GM) in agriculture.

One of the key disputes in the debate on legislative reforms dealing with GM is whether strict legal liability should be imposed on the manufacturers of GM products, such as seeds.[14] Strict liability would not require the manufacturer to be negligent in order to be liable for damages—it would only be necessary that the product be defective and dangerous to use. This does not make strict liability a compensation automate, but reduces the burden of proof of the claimant as compared to, for instance, damages sought on the basis of negligence.

In law, strict liability is closely associated with general products liability: that is, liability for manufactured goods and, more recently, for services and intangibles. In most jurisdictions, products liability is taken in terms of strict liability—either in written law or in common law. This is not yet the case with GM. In common law countries there have not been enough tried cases of GM damages for a legal standpoint to have become established, and elsewhere, most notably in Europe, only Austria and Germany have strict liability legal regimes applying to GM.

The New Zealand Royal Commission on Genetic Modification has produced a report that contains extensive coverage of the international debate and legislation on GM. The report concludes that the common law has adequate measures to handle the liability issue. This does not exhaust the option that strict liability will prevail, but will leave it dependent on judges' verdicts. However, the fundamental reason why the Commission did not advocate written law imposing strict liability is evident in its view that the use of strict liability would be a barrier to innovation and progress.[15] Similar reasoning has taken the upper hand in the United States, where GM is not officially recognized as an environmental hazard. As a consequence, it has become more risky for potential claimants to take GM corporations to court for damages, as the claimants would have to establish the inherent hazardousness of GM in order to be successful. This is in sharp contrast to the policy adopted in Europe. In the European Union's directive proposal for Environmental Liability, GM is subject to a special legal regime providing for a wide range of strict liability areas.[16]

So, we have conflicting views about what kind of legal regime should prevail. It is a classic case on which ethical considerations can be brought to bear. In whose favor would stakeholder value philosophy turn the scales? Such a philosophy emphasizes that the corporation is ethically responsible to all its stakeholders. So, a manufacturer of GM seeds is responsible for the damages they cause; but to what extent responsible? Is negligence required, or should the manufacturer consider GM products as inherently dangerous and exercise appropriate caution before entering the market?

Here we have no need to go into the largely unresolved disputes of the hazardousness of GM products. As philosophers, we may be content with less contested propositions, like "a product is a product is a product." In other words, modern law includes under the concept of "product" not only manufactured goods, but also a wide array of services and intangibles. Against this background it is quite hard to justify the suggestion that GM agricultural product is not a product. Therefore, we have, *prima facie*, no reason to treat GM products differently from other products falling under the strict liability regime.

Stakeholder value is a forceful ethical argument establishing a moral relation between the manufacturer of goods and the customers who purchase those goods. Law already widely recognizes that this moral relation entails strict liability, which means that it is the manufacturers' duty to make sure that the products do not carry an unreasonable risk. From the point of view of stakeholder ethics, nothing suggests that the situation should be different in the case of GM products.

New Zealand Law Commission's reason for not advocating strict liability in written law reveals that tougher financial liability would increase the cost and risks of GM research, making companies more careful before they launch new GM products. From the viewpoint of stakeholder ethics, this outcome from strict liability sounds like a most desirable one. It would improve corporate deliberation, and most probably also the standards of products sold. At the same time it would be in accordance with the spirit of market economy by leaving the risk assessment to corporations themselves, with the chance that they make money if they choose correctly, but pay if their judgment falters.

I conclude by suggesting that the above line of argument is applicable to other fields of bioethics and medical ethics as well. The issues may there be even more loaded with passions and emotions, but the fundamental structure of ethical problems carries many similarities to the GM case. Take artificial insemination or human cloning. The first is already big business, the second is at least in a start-up phase of its business cycle. I do not wish to say that human cloning should be made legal. There may well be plenty of reasons that it should not. But what could, at least, be concluded from stakeholder value business ethics is that strict liability should apply to the producers of cloning or in vitro fertilization services. If the service is to produce a human being, the service provider should, from the standpoint of rational ethics, be held as responsible for the life created as any other agent creating life. Whether the decisions that bring about the child are made in a boardroom or inside a person's body and mind, and regardless of the medium employed being a test-tube or muscular and mucosal contact, the ethical implications as to the well-being of the life created should be the same.

Stakeholder value philosophy shows that issues in bioethics can be solved by examining business'—inherently very ethical—character. In bioethics it backs strict products liability, which in more conventional fields of production is already a broadly applied and accepted measure to erect efficient market controls against potentially hazardous technologies without affecting markets' basic dynamics. If financial gain is sought in biotechnology or medicine, the best deterrent against unethical activity may well be financial liability instead of prohibition.

8. Competition and the Moral of Markets

The outcome of a philosophical analysis of corporate ethical responsibility is that even if we begin with the view—shared by economics, anthropology, and jurisprudence—of the corporation as a contractual medium of rationally self-interested individuals, designed to advance those individuals' well-being, we can show that this corporate medium is a bearer of ethical responsibilities, rights, and duties.

It is not necessary to introduce ethics into business from sources external to business itself, for instance from the idealistic and altruistic concept of the virtuous self propounded by virtue ethics. Business is naturally infused with ethics. Trust, honesty, and equality of opportunity are necessary conditions of good business—and even more, they are necessary conditions of any well-functioning, competitive market. This fact has encouraged the crusader of stakeholder philosophy, Thomas Donaldson, to speak of the ethical advantage of nations, analogous to Harvard economist Michael Porter's famous idea of the competitive advantage of nations based on their ability to innovate.[17] An example supporting Donaldson's thesis of competitive advantage provided by ethics could be the global success of Nokia, and some other lesser-known Finnish companies. Without underestimating the skills of Finns in technology and commerce, it can be suggested that their winning streaks are partly founded on high standards in business ethics: they are known as reliable, uncorrupted business partners, and these qualities attract partners and clients.

However, the ethics of a competitive market economy has a reach deeper than mere ethical business practices and the respect of the interests of all stakeholders. Markets entail freedom of action that respects autonomy as a fundamental trait of human nature; efficiency that creates the maximum amount of welfare out of given limited resources; and competition that eliminates surplus profits. In addition, business is universal: in aiming at profit, it treats everybody equally regardless of nationality, race, or religion. It is an activity that promotes social interaction between people, political stability, democracy, and peace, without which no business can survive and succeed in the long run.

To sum up, business contains, both on the macro-level as a competitive market economy and on the micro-level as a corporation, plenty of elements which most ethical theories would assess as good, or right, or desirable. Against this background it is a hollow claim that business should adopt an altruistic ethical standard from outside the commercial activity itself. The claim is also paradoxical because it goes directly against the fundamental logics and benefits of a competitive market: as a matter of fact, monopolies would have the best resources for altruistic charity—companies competing in an efficient market have very low margins for that end.

The fundamental social function of business is the efficient production of goods and services. In carrying out this function, businesses harness the rational self-interestedness of individuals to service the common good. Corporate ethical responsibility facilitates this process by presuming respect for the legal framework erected by democratic government—including laws implementing income redistribution—and respect for the interests of all stakeholders of the corporation.

The corporation may take heed of its ethical responsibility in its organization by implementing a wide array of means and practices. Examples are improvements in corporate governance, channels to promote interaction between stakeholder groups, codes of ethics, training, and ethical auditing. All these measures, and many others aiming at the same end, are already routine in thousands of companies, especially in the United States. They are concrete expressions of the fact that "business ethics" is no oxymoron. On the contrary, good business is infused by ethics, and business ethics is the area of philosophy dealing with values of business and business problems related to values.[18]

NOTES

1. Aristotle, *The Politics*, trans. T. A. Sinclair (Bungay, Suffolk: Penguin Books, 1979), p. 46. See also Norman Barry, *Business Ethics* (London: Macmillan Press Ltd), 1998.

2. James Gordley, *The Philosophical Origins of Modern Contract Doctrine* (New York, NY: Oxford University Press, 1991).

3. G. H. von Wright, *The Varieties of Goodness* (London: Routledge and Kegan Paul, 1963).

4. See Michael Smith, *The Moral Problem* (Oxford: Blackwell, 1994).

5. See *The Ethics of Aristotle. The Nicomachean Ethics*, trans. J. A. K. Thomson (Aylesbury: Penguin Books, 1976), pp. 219–220.

6. Jonathan Jacobs, "Metaethics and Teleology," *The Review of Metaphysics*, 55:1 (September 2001), pp. 50–51.

7. Barry, *Business Ethics.*

8. Milton Friedman, "The Social Responsibility of Business is to Increase its Profits," *Business Ethics: A Philosophical Reader*, ed. T. I. White (New York: Macmillan, 1993), pp. 162–167.

9. Peter A. French, "The Corporation as a Moral Person," *Business Ethics: A Philosophical Reader*, ed. T. I. White (New York, NY: Macmillan, 1993), pp. 167–187.

10. See, for instance Thomas Donaldson, "Constructing a Social Contract for Business," *Business Ethics*, ed. T. I. White, pp. 167–187; Kenneth E. Goodpaster, "Business Ethics and Stakeholder Analysis," *Business Ethics*, ed. T. I. White, pp. 205–223; Patricia Werhane, *Persons, Rights, and Corporations* (Englewood Cliffs, NJ: Prentice-Hall, 1985).

11. E. F. Fama, "Agency Problems and the Theory of the Firm," *Journal of Political Economy*, 88:2 (1980), pp. 288–307.

12. D. Millon, "Theories of the Corporation," *Duke Law Journal* (1990), pp. 201–262.

13. C. Fried, *Contract as Promise* (Cambridge, MA: Harvard University Press, 1981).

14. See D. L. Kershen, "An Agricultural Law Research Article: Legal Liability Issues in Agricultural Biotechnology," http://www.nationalaglawcenter.org.

15. *Royal Commission on Genetic Modification Report*, www.gmcommission.
govt.nz, p. 328.

16. Kershen, "An Agricultural Law Research Article," p. 4.

17. Thomas Donaldson, "The Ethical Wealth of Nations," *Journal of Business Ethics*, 31 (2001), pp. 25–36.

18. I am indebted to Matti Häyry and Peter Herissone-Kelly for their comments on earlier drafts of this paper.

Eleven

PERSPECTIVISM IN RISK MANAGEMENT

Peter Lucas

1. Introduction

The debate concerning the use of economic appraisal methods such as cost-benefit analysis (CBA) in healthcare decision making has now extended over several decades.[1] Arguing in favor of the use of such methods, economists have pointed out that they represent a straightforward means by which healthcare workers can fulfill their ethical obligation to ensure that limited resources are used with maximum efficiency.[2] Opposition to the use of economic appraisal methods has tended to take one of two forms. First, it has been argued that something in the economic approach to healthcare decision making is essentially incompatible with traditional medical ethics. Second, attention has focused on difficulties confronting the use of economic methods in practice: for example, the difficulty of developing suitable measures of health. The use of non-monetary measures of health such as the "Quality Adjusted Life Year" (QALY) has excited particular controversy.[3]

In the midst of all this, comparatively little attention seems to have been paid to the question of the general defensibility of the use of CBA and CBA-inspired methods as decision making guides in healthcare contexts. Indeed, we might easily be forgiven for thinking that the method itself is essentially problem free, and that any difficulties associated with it arise more from the conditions of its use than from anything inherent in it. The present paper aims to challenge such a view. I shall argue that, for reasons having to do with the ineradicable uncertainty afflicting all healthcare decision making, economic appraisal methods such as CBA are essentially unsuitable in a wide range of healthcare contexts. The apparent legitimacy of the use of economic appraisal methods in contexts of uncertainty derives, as we shall see, from the apparent plausibility of the assumption that rational risk management essentially involves the maximization of expected net utility. But the latter assumption is by no means as safe as it may initially appear.

The main piece of evidence I shall cite against this assumption is the existence of the insurance industry—or, more precisely, the existence of insurance agreements that may be rationally entered into by both contracting parties. The existence of such agreements, I will argue, reveals that risk management is an inherently perspectival (or, if you prefer, "contextual") affair: there may be a multitude of equally rational perspectives on the same risk, and the perspective according to which the rational response to a given risk involves the maximization of expected net utility may be only one among a range of rational responses to that risk, if it falls within that range at all.

My argument in what follows has most relevance to those healthcare decision making contexts directly affected by the rise of economic methods—for example, to questions of resource allocation.[4] However, if it is sound, the argument will also have broader application. The view that rational risk management essentially involves the maximization of expected net utility is also held by many ethical consequentialists, who may otherwise have little in common with the proponents of economic appraisal (not least because of the sheer variety of ways in which "utility" is understood—for example as preference satisfaction, interest satisfaction, or "welfare" in the economist's sense—the satisfaction of preferences expressed through market choices). While my explicit focus is relatively narrow then—the question of the defensibility of the use of economic appraisal methods in healthcare contexts subject to significant uncertainty—the argument also has implications for the general defensibility of consequentialist decision making in contexts of uncertainty.

2. Economic Decision Making and Risk Neutrality

In practice, all healthcare decision making involves an element of uncertainty. Healthcare institutions, medical procedures, and the human body being as they inevitably are, we can never be entirely sure that what emerges at the culmination of any decision making process as the preferred option will subsequently be realized in practice. Strictly speaking, we are always working in the realm of probabilities, rather than certainties. Of course, it is as easy to overstate the extent of our uncertainty as to understate it. In many circumstances the extent of any relevant uncertainty will be minimal, and may perhaps be legitimately ignored. But in many other cases this will not be the case. In this chapter I shall be concerned to highlight problems that arise in connection with the use of economic appraisal methods such as CBA (and its derivatives) in contexts marked by *significant* uncertainty. (To specify more precisely which types of contexts are marked by significant uncertainty goes beyond the scope of this chapter. I shall proceed on the assumption that such cases exist, and that they form a significant proportion of the total range of contexts in which healthcare decisions are made.) I shall argue that economic methods are unsuitable in cases involving significant uncertainty, and that their use in such cases will only serve to preempt, if not obstruct, more properly deliberative decision making processes.

Economic decision making methods evaluate the different alternative options in any given decision making context according to the relative contributions they promise to make to aggregate levels of human welfare, measured in terms of the satisfaction of individual preferences. The course of action to be preferred is that which promises to deliver the highest benefit-cost ratio, maximizing expected net utility. There are several variants of the basic benefit-cost model, the choice between which will depend on whether the options available can plausibly be assigned monetary values, and whether the calculation is intended to take account of economic externalities.[5] Defending the general legitimacy of such approaches, their proponents typically appeal to their alleged rationality: "[A] rational *social decision* is one in which the benefits to society (i.e. the sum of people in society) exceed the costs."[6]

In order to maximize expected utility in contexts of significant uncertainty however, such economic decision making methods must be allied to an attitude of strict *risk neutrality*. Economists concerned with the descriptive analytics of risk standardly distinguish three different attitudes to risk, under the headings of "risk aversion," "risk neutrality," and "risk preference."[7] We can bring out the distinctive characters of these attitudes by considering how representatives of each would tend to view the adage that "a bird in the hand is worth two in the bush."

Other things being equal (and assuming for present purposes the homogeneity and general desirability of members of the class of "birds"), we would expect a risk neutral individual to agree that a bird in the hand is worth two in the bush where and only where the odds of retrieval of any one bird from the bush are 0.5. If the odds of retrieval of the birds from the bush were significantly greater than 0.5, then a risk neutral individual would be inclined to take a chance on the two in the bush, rather than cling to the bird in hand. On the other hand, where the odds of retrieval of each were significantly less than 0.5 a risk neutral individual would prefer the bird in the hand. Risk averse individuals by contrast would tend to prefer the bird in the hand even for odds of retrieval of the birds in the bush significantly higher than 0.5. Despite the fact that, at odds of retrieval of 0.6, the goal of maximizing expected net utility would be best served by relinquishing the bird in hand for a chance at the two in the bush, the risk averse individual would prefer to pass up this opportunity, and cling to the security represented by the bird in the hand. Risk preferring individuals would be inclined to depart from risk neutrality in the opposite direction. A risk preferring individual would be prepared to relinquish the bird in the hand for a chance at the two in the bush even at odds of retrieval for each of significantly less than 0.5.

It follows that both risk averse and risk preferring individuals will regularly make decisions that fail to maximize expected net utility—risk averse individuals failing to capitalize on good opportunities to increase net utility, risk preferring individuals rashly risking secure assets in what (to a risk neutral individual at least) would appear to be a misguided attempt to add to those assets.

Given that both risk aversion and risk preference are associated with behavior that fails to maximize expected net utility, it is evident that enthusiasts for economic decision making methods must, in contexts of significant uncertainty, eschew both attitudes, and preserve instead an attitude of strict risk neutrality. Nevertheless, as I will now explain, in many cases an attitude of risk neutrality is by no means the key to the rational management of risk.

3. Risk Neutrality and Rationality

The thought that an attitude of risk neutrality is essential to rational risk management might seem to receive support from examples such as that of a casino operator, whose guiding principle is to accept any bet so long as the balance of the odds and the sums at stake come out in the house's favor. Such a principle combines prudence with respect to existing assets, with an appropriate boldness where opportunities exist to increase those assets. Strict adherence to the principle might well see the casino operator through a run of bad luck. Imagine a case in which a customer hits a winning streak, repeatedly betting successfully, against all the odds. In a case like this the casino operator is virtually assured of a profit in the long run as long as she keeps doggedly on taking the customer's bets. Indeed, in such a case we might well contrast the (perhaps) irrational emotional state of the customer, who proves unable to leave the table during her winning streak, with the steady confidence of the casino owner in the face of short term setbacks: "in the long run, if the odds are right, I cannot lose."

In the light of such examples it may be tempting to take such risk neutral conduct as our paradigm of rational risk management. To do so, however, would be a mistake. It simply is not the case that an attitude of strict risk neutrality is the key to rational risk management, even for someone in the position of a casino operator. Suppose a customer were to come into the casino and place a massive bet, at long odds, such that if she were to win the casino would be bankrupted. Should the casino operator take the bet? Reason may well say "No." Even in a case in which the bet is a poor one from the customer's point of view—that is, where the ratios of stake to potential payout, in the light of the odds, are such that only a risk preferring individual would willingly place such a bet—the possibility of catastrophic loss for the casino will still be there. And in such circumstances the risk neutral path, and the path of prudence, may well diverge. While at a superficial level the rational response for the casino operator may look to be that of taking the bet, she must also take into account the potentially catastrophic consequences of losing, unlikely though losing may be. Adopting a risk neutral attitude in this case may well be a luxury the casino operator cannot afford. Instead, the prudent course might well be to pass up what remains in principle a good opportunity to turn a profit, on the basis that the prospects should the customer win are, from the casino's perspective, too appalling to contemplate.

It is evident, then, that in at least some cases those whose commercial interests are generally best served by maintaining an attitude of risk neutrality must depart from the principle of taking any bet so long as the ratio of odds to potential payout are favorable. When the absolute levels of stake and potential payout rise too high, an ideal of risk neutrality is no longer a reliable guide. The rational response to some risks is an attitude of risk aversion.

Equally, the casino operator may sometimes rationally depart from an attitude of risk neutrality in the opposite direction: that of risk preference. There is, for example, no obvious reason why the casino operator should not play the national lottery. The odds against a win might be astronomical, but the prize is fabulous, and the ticket price is (for most of us) negligible. Despite the fact that, the odds against success being so huge, a bet on the national lottery is of a type that, generally speaking, only a risk preferring individual would willingly make, there remains, for many of us, nothing obviously irrational in playing the national lottery. Where we have an opportunity to stake an insignificant amount on a chance of winning millions, albeit at extremely long odds, risk preference may well make more sense than risk neutrality.

On closer inspection then, the case of the casino operator reveals that if there is a connection between risk neutrality and rational risk management, it is a more complicated connection than might have at first appeared. For the casino operator, risk neutrality only makes sense within certain limits, and these limits will be determined by such contextual factors as the extent of the financial reserves available. There will be many cases in which a struggling concern will (rationally) adopt an attitude of risk aversion where a well-resourced competitor would (rationally) have taken the bet.

However, perhaps the best illustration of the limits of the view that equates rational risk management with the maintenance of an attitude of risk neutrality, and thus with the maximization of expected net utility, is provided by the insurance industry. The barroom economist, who simplistically equates rational risk management with the maintenance of an attitude of risk neutrality, and on that basis argues that it is irrational to take out insurance (since we are always likely to pay out more in premiums than we will recoup in payouts), will be a familiar figure to many. Here again, though, what promises to be the most profitable course is not always the most rational course. When, for example, I insure my home against fire, I am insuring what I cannot afford to replace. Consequently, I have compelling rational grounds for risk aversion in this case. Statistically speaking, it may be a "good" bet that my house will not burn down. Nevertheless, it is not a good bet from my point of view. Just as the casino operator may well find herself in situations in which it will not make sense to take what, from some other possible perspectives, looks like a "good" bet, so in our lives there are many cases in which the chances of loss are extremely low, but the consequences of losing are catastrophic; and in these cases an attitude of risk aversion will usually be the rational response. It may be in some sense a "good" bet that my house will not burn down. But it remains a risk I ought to buy out of, if I can.

When I buy insurance my insurer shoulders, for a price, the risk I cannot afford to remain exposed to. If I have rationally sought such protection, does it follow that it is irrational of my insurer to take on the risk exposure on my behalf? Not necessarily. A vast proportion of my total assets are tied up in my house. For my insurer, on the other hand, the value of my house represents a drop in the ocean of her total assets. The risk associated with my house burning down is therefore a risk with respect to which she can afford to remain sanguine. My insurer can rationally maintain an attitude of risk neutrality in cases in which the rational response for me is one of risk aversion, and it is this difference of perspective that explains how it is that both parties can rationally enter into the insurance contract: the insurer can rationally take on exposure to a risk that the insuree rationally buys protection from.

It is important to note that in such cases it is perfectly possible that both parties to the contract will agree on every quantifiable detail of the risk in question. In the case I have mentioned, my insurer and I might well agree (though we need not) on the value of my house, the value of my yearly premium, and the odds of my house being destroyed by fire. That my insurer will rationally take on exposure to a risk that I rationally buy protection from does not necessarily reflect a difference in our estimation of the *nature* of the risk. The crucial difference, which serves to make it possible for both parties to rationally enter into the contract, may simply be that—with her vast financial reserves—the insurer is in a position rationally to maintain an attitude of risk neutrality in cases in which the insuree is not.

4. Perspectivism and Risk

In recent years a good deal of attention has been paid to the question whether risk is "objective"—by which is usually meant something like "open to precise and impartial quantification," or "subjective"—by which is usually meant something like "fundamentally dependent on psychological/cultural filters."[8] What the insurance example reveals however is that the question whether risk is objective or subjective does not represent the most helpful framing of the issues. The insurance example shows that rational risk management is a thoroughly perspectival (or again, if you prefer, "contextual") affair. Even when all the quantifiable facts concerning a given risk are in, there remains the question whether those exposed to that risk can rationally view their risk exposure with equanimity, or would be better advised to seek risk protection, and equally whether some of those not exposed to that risk might be well advised to take on more risk exposure—for a fee. In neither case can we afford to assume that a model that considers risk neutrality to be the key to rational risk management will prove a reliable guide.

So there is no need to invoke controversial claims about the role of cultural filters to highlight the shortcomings of an "objectivist" approach to understanding risk. Even if we grant, for argument's sake, central objectivist assumptions regarding the quantifiability of risks: that it is possible to produce reliable (monetary or non-monetary) measures of potential costs and benefits, and to establish with reasonable accuracy the odds that various alternative outcomes will occur; that there is no single rational attitude to risk—that risk neutrality, risk aversion and even risk preference may each represent a rational response to a specific risk in specific circumstances—indicates that the objectivist account tells only part of the story. (The insurance example also has the merit of showing that risk aversion can be a rational response to risk exposure in many more mundane cases than our casino example might suggest.)

Moreover, just what the objectivist account leaves out looks like an indispensable part of the story, for decision making purposes. If risk aversion and risk preference are rational responses to risk in some circumstances, the apparent justification for the indiscriminate use of economic decision making methods in risk contexts collapses. As we have seen, the use of such methods appears legitimate only where they are allied to an attitude of strict risk neutrality. The claim is that such methods represent the key to rational decision making because they maximize expected net utility. But as we have also seen, there are a huge number of mundane cases in which the ideal of maximizing expected net utility does not represent the key to rational risk management. In these cases, economic methods will, as a result of their intrinsic link to the risk neutral perspective—from which they cannot be divorced without losing touch with their legitimizing ground—be a patently *un*reliable guide to rational decision making. It appears then that in all but the most trivial cases the question whether the goal of maximizing expected utility is appropriate to a given decision making context cannot be satisfactorily answered without considering the host of contextual factors which may entail that an attitude of risk aversion (or risk preference) will be the more rational response.

There are several means by which decision making processes might be designed to take account of the contextual factors I have mentioned, to which I can only gesture briefly here. Perhaps the most important distinction amongst these means lies between those that hinge on the outcome of some expert inquiry into the context in question, and those that strive, in varying degrees, and by varying methods, to build some lay involvement into the process. The false promise of economic methods rested on the fact that while they appear to offer a short cut to rational risk management, they actually exclude a crucial segment of the data that rational risk management depends upon: contextual information regarding who is exposed to risk, and how important the items at risk are to them (such "importance" is not the same thing as "economic value," since for many people items of relatively little economic value are nevertheless of enormous worth). Genuinely rational risk management processes would take into account not only the economic value of the items at risk, but also whether the loss of those items would represent a catastrophe for those affected. Indeed it is part of the pathos of many decision dilemmas in healthcare and elsewhere that they involve cases of actual and potential personal catastrophes, whose economic costs are trivial. The proper response to such cases is not simply to protest that we cannot put an accurate economic value on the cost of these catastrophes (though this may well be true), but to insist in addition that economic measures do not tell us what we really need to know: whether the costs in question are costs which those affected can afford to pay.

It is not unthinkable that an expert-driven approach to understanding risk, which found a way to take the contextual factors I have adverted to properly into account, would qualify as a satisfactory alternative to the use of economic methods. What is most obviously wrong with the use of economic methods in risk contexts is not that they are "expert-driven," but that they attempt to base decision making on inappropriate short cuts. That said, it appears likely that the most politically acceptable alternatives to the use of economic methods will display limited dependence on expert knowledge, and provide significant scope for lay involvement. In establishing how, precisely, we should take account of the various contextual factors that jointly determine whether a given potential cost is one that an individual or group of individuals can rationally accept exposure to, it does not seem unreasonable to suggest that the individuals involved should be consulted directly. Having accepted the principle of direct lay involvement, however, several routes lie open to us. These range from straightforward polling methods, to the host of techniques associated with deliberative democratic procedures. My own predilections and commitments would lead me to favor the second class of alternatives. Be that as it may, my main goal in this chapter has been firstly that of showing that economic decision making methods are not a universally reliable guide to rational decision making, and secondly that of indicating where their primary shortcomings lie.

NOTES

1. See e.g. J. A. Gray, "Choosing Priorities," *Journal of Medical Ethics*, 5 (June 1979), pp. 73–74; Gavin Mooney, *Economics, Medicine, and Healthcare* (Hemel Hempstead: Harvester, 2nd ed., 1992). For an overview of ethical issues see Tom L. Beauchamp and James F. Childress *Principles of Biomedical Ethics* (Oxford: Oxford University Press, 5th ed., 2001), pp. 194–214. For a recent perspective from economics see Paul McCrone, *Understanding Health Economics* (London: Kogan Page, 1998), Introduction. For a critical sociological view

see Malcolm Ashmore, Michael Mulkay, and Trevor Pinch, *Health and Efficiency: A Sociology of Health Economics* (Milton Keynes: Open University Press, 1989).

2. See Mooney, *Economics, Medicine, and Healthcare.*

3. See Beauchamp and Childress, *Principles of Biomedical Ethics*, pp. 206–214.

4. See *ibid.*, pp. 250–272.

5. See McCrone, *Understanding Health Economics*, chapters 3 and 5.

6. David Pearce, *Cost-Benefit Analysis* (London: Macmillan, 2nd ed., 1983), p. 3.

7. See e.g. Jack Hirshleifer and John Riley, *The Analytics of Uncertainty and Information* (Cambridge: Cambridge University Press, 1992).

8. For a useful summary of views see Sheila Jasanoff, "The Songlines of Risk," *Environmental Values*, 8:2 (May 1999), pp. 135–52.

Twelve

MORAL PROGRESS

Simon Woods

1. Introduction

In this chapter I will make an argument, albeit a rather intuitive argument, in support of moral progress. Having tested various versions of this argument at various times and with quite diverse audiences, and almost always found a stubborn degree of objection to this claim, I can only anticipate a similar response in the reader. There are in fact two sorts of claim involved in this argument, and most audiences give a grudging acceptance to the weaker claim that we can at least make sense of the possibility of moral progress, but respond with an almost universal rejection of the stronger claim that we have undergone moral progress. I would not be surprised if the reader has a similar reaction. This seems all the more reasonable given that I am writing this in the post-Bosnia, post-Rwanda, post-11 September era, and in the midst of the second Gulf War. Our inhumanity to each other and our moral myopathy are daily flashed across the world courtesy of the contemporaneous coverage the modern media provide. The reasons I would give the reader for persisting with this paper can be established by taking a moment for some Cartesian reflection. What, you should ask yourself, are the consequences of denying either of the claims I make? I would suggest that the consequences are not only deeply counterintuitive, but also profoundly pessimistic. There is of course an alternative view—namely, that it is not the claims that are false, but my defense of the claims that is inadequate. But to come to this conclusion you will have to consider the arguments—so read on!

2. Moral Progress

As an applied philosopher working in the field of bioethics, most of my time is spent teaching ethics to health workers. It seems to me that this would be a task of Sisyphean pointlessness if there were not at least the possibility of moral progress. The very reason for teaching ethics to healthcare workers is not merely to acquaint them with moral theory or the history of philosophy, but to enable them to recognize the moral dimension to their work, and, by incorporating practical moral reasoning into the process of making clinical judgments, to make *better* judgments. Also—and I believe that this is not too grandiose a claim—individuals might become better doctors, nurses, and therapists, and perhaps even better people.

This is not to say that a commitment to moral progress is equivalent to the belief that we are, as Condorcet puts it "advancing with a firm and sure step along the path of truth, virtue, and happiness."[1] It is a strange anomaly that though there is moral progress, this does not entail that the world is always and everywhere a better place—but more on this later. First I want to say something about the metaphysics of progress.

In order to understand moral progress, we need a conception of progress that is adequate to the task. One conception of progress is as a species of change. And to understand change we need an understanding of the relative parameters by which a thing may be judged to have changed. The metaphysical arguments are complex, and this short chapter does not allow for the detailed discussion required, so I shall use the opportunity to develop my argument at a more intuitive level.

3. Progress and Change

Take the progress of a train along a track as an example of change. A simple way of describing the train's progress is in terms of its change in position relative to stationary objects over time. So one set of possible parameters of progress consists of the different spatio-temporal co-ordinates of the object in question, which are useful in this case for measuring the train's progress along the track. The train's progress can therefore be represented in terms of the difference between our observations of the train at time 1 (t_1) and position 1 (p_1) compared to the observations at t_2 and p_2. One way in which this account of progress may have an analogy in terms of moral progress is to consider the temporal aspect: that progress is a function of change over time. However, in terms of moral progress this seems inadequate, for whilst the temporal co-ordinates may apply, since it takes at least two reference points to make a comparison possible, what are the moral equivalents of the spatial co-ordinates? There are of course some possible candidates: for example, the claim that at t_1 slavery is widely practiced, while at t_2 slavery is not widely practiced seems to have the same form as our account of the train's progress. The problem with this example is that we are unable to distinguish between putative moral progress and the mere reporting of a difference over time, which may be a non-moral difference or even a report of moral regress, without some further account of why this is *moral* progress rather than a report of a mere change. A possible solution to consider is the idea that progress is a form of teleological change, so that progress may be judged relative to the goal or end aimed at. Applying the teleological concept to the train example seems to give a more meaningful account of the train's progress if we consider that progress as more purposeful than a mere change in position, so that, for example, the progress of the train is measured relative to the station to which it is traveling.

So does the addition of teleological considerations represent an improved model of moral progress? If anything, introducing teleological considerations adds a further tier of complexity to the notion of moral progress. On one level such an account seems to create a demand for an impossibly realist account of morality on a Platonic scale. On this account we would already need to know the "good"—to know where we are going in the first place—in order to make the judgment that a change constitutes progress. But the nature of the "good" is the very thing contested in moral disputes. A skeptic might observe that any candidate for a good will always be radically underdetermined by the different and competing accounts of that good offered by different agents. This kind of teleological account is impossibly demanding if it requires that we have infallible knowledge of the "good" before we are able to work out our progress in relation to particular moral problems. This is not the account of moral progress I have in mind, although I do believe that a form of teleological account is appropriate.

The account I have in mind is not one that entails ontological claims on the grand scale, but is rather an account of moral epistemology, the process of practical moral reasoning, and the objectivity of judgment in relation to the goals of morality. What are the goals of morality? Well, consistent with my account above, I do not believe that we have anything approaching an exhaustive account of such goals or ends, but that does not mean that we have no account at all. Human experience has furnished us with knowledge enough to begin to shade in, and shade in with quite some detail, some of the general concepts, such as flourishing or equal respect, that otherwise sound good but seem empty. There is a useful, if cautiously drawn, analogy here with knowledge in the context of the natural sciences. The lack of a Grand Unifying Theory, or our lack of a complete knowledge of matter, does not undermine the ability of the natural sciences to provide "good enough" explanations of the physical world, nor does it mean that endeavors to seek such a theory, or pursue such knowledge, are not useful and important enterprises. I do not believe that moral philosophy is concerned with uncovering new moral "facts," but that it is concerned with the deepening and enriching of our moral understanding.

To claim that there are such goals and goods as flourishing and equality does not require us to give a substantive account of them in advance, since the process of shading in the detail of such goals, the process of rejecting or accepting different accounts of them, is itself a process by which our understanding is deepened and enriched. Charles Taylor talks of such moral postulates as "hypergoods, i.e., goods which are not only incomparably more important than others but provide the standpoint from which these must be weighed, judged, decided about."[2] The process of reflective deliberation is one by which it is possible to come to the judgment that one course of action or another—one conjectured account of the good over another—is superior. It is a process repeated and echoed at many levels, from individual introspections to more collective deliberations, a process by which a new nuance or layer of insight can be brought to moral understanding. The questioning and challenging of the established boundaries of certain moral concepts has in many cases advanced the "baseline," or extended the boundary, to the extent that the new parameter is at least the presumed position from which we start, in terms of personal behavior and the values that underpin wider social institutions.[3] This is not to say that progress is inevitable, but minimally, as Thomas Nagel comments, that progress starts with something's having become established as "obvious," and our setting out from there.[4]

An example of this "point of departure approach" is reflected in the altered view regarding the set of entities to which notions of equal respect apply. This has been irreversibly expanded from a position from which women were unquestionably excluded, to the position where women are unquestionably included, or at least the presumption is that those who continue to exclude women need to argue their case against where the boundary is now set.

Although the boundaries of equal respect have been extended in one direction to the point where contraction is almost inconceivable, the boundaries are not immutable. The frontiers of contemporary moral debate are characterized by disputes as to whether the boundaries can be redrawn in a way that constitutes a superior set of discriminations, for example whether notions of equal respect can be meaningfully expanded to, say, non-human animals on the one hand, and contracted to exclude the human "non-person" on the other.[5]

The process of this discourse echoes Charles Taylor's account of the ranking of different goods based on the "epistemic gain" of the proffered solution: "We are convinced that a certain view is superior because we have lived a transition which we understand as error-reducing and hence as epistemic gain."[6]

4. Ameliorative Change

The idea that a necessary component of moral progress is a sense of things improving has led Stan Godlovitch to reject teleological change as a model for moral progress, in favor of an account of ameliorative change. Godlovitch suggests that we can judge such progress with the benefit of retrospective evaluation—"things look better from here considering where we've just come from."[7] Retrospective evaluation is of course only one form of comparison that contributes to the general idea of moral progress. The comparison of the moral status of slavery at different times, for example, must amount to more than a simple observation on the *practice* of slavery, if it is to count as a claim for moral progress. This is because a report that slavery is no longer widely practiced leaves open the question of the moral status of slavery. If this observation is also a claim for moral progress, then there must be an appeal to a specifically moral claim that slavery is wrong. To be convinced by this we must look not only to the robustness of our arguments, but also to the way in which this claim coheres with the rest of moral knowledge. A claim about the wrongness of slavery implies that we have also, at least partially, worked out what is meant by such concepts as "liberty," "equality," and the moral status of "persons," to name but a few. The notion of moral progress is therefore not only evident in retrospective evaluations, but in the very possibility of moral argument itself.

So the idea that ameliorative change can only be judged with the benefit of hindsight is not the whole story. A judgment of moral progress, a judgment that one moral claim is better than another, need not entail a comparison over time but could equally, and indeed often is, made by standing competing moral claims side by side. This is not to say that our judgments of moral progress are entirely abstract affairs involving reason alone, for we must have knowledge of human harm and suffering to give substance to our moral concepts. A number of different aspects are involved when making the judgment that one moral claim is an improvement upon another. One of these is moral relevance—a good judgment is one that is sensitive to whether different properties are morally relevant or not. Progress has been made in moral discourse by showing that age, color, and even species are not morally relevant in the way they were once assumed to be when deciding between the different interests of competing individuals or groups. Another example concerns judgments regarding the most appropriate "fit" of our moral concepts, or what I call "moral extension." Moral progress can be judged in terms of the way in which a moral category has been extended to become more inclusive—less discriminatory in one sense and more discriminating in another—as I have suggested with the example of equal respect.

This marks the end of the preamble. I now turn to the more applied approach, in which I first present an account of *personal* moral progress, and then go on to argue that this account is a useful, and indeed a robust, model for understanding moral progress in general.

5. Personal Moral Progress

My account of personal moral progress relies upon an extended thought experiment, and therefore requires some participation from the reader. The following section is an extract from Charles Dickens's novel *Martin Chuzzlewit*.[8] I suggest that for the first task in this practical exercise you read and enjoy this extract. For readers who are not familiar with Dickens's novel, the following points will set the scene. Mrs Gamp, referred to in the text as a "nurse," has been hired, with her colleague Mrs Prig, to share the care of a "John Doe" patient, a young man, identity unknown, who is delirious with fever. The reader enters the scene at the point where Mrs Prig is handing over the care of the patient to Mrs Gamp who will be in attendance during the night. This extract is my own abridgement, and I would encourage the reader to read the whole of the chapter for the full effect.

> She had begun to make signs of inquiry in reference to the position of the patient and his overhearing them … when Mrs Prig settled that point easily.
>
> "Oh!" she said aloud, "he's quiet, but his wits is gone. It an't no matter wot you say."
>
> "Anythin' to tell afore you goes, my dear?" asked Mrs Gamp, setting her bundle down inside the door, and looking affectionately at her partner.

Mrs Prig merely comments on the quality of the food available for the "carers" and adds as an afterthought:

> "The physic and them things is on the drawers and mankleshelf," said Mrs Prig, cursorily. "He took his last slime draught at seven. The easy-chair an't soft enough. You'll want his piller."
>
> Mrs Gamp thanked her for these hints, and giving her a friendly good night, held the door open until she had disappeared at the other end of the gallery. Having thus performed the hospitable duty of seeing her safely off, she shut it, locked it on the inside, took up her bundle, walked round the screen, and entered on her occupation of the sick chamber.

The first thing Mrs Gamp does is to examine the accommodation with a view to her own comfort before turning to examine the patient.

> Mrs Gamp solaced herself with a pinch of snuff, and stood looking at him with her head inclined a little sideways, as a connoisseur might gaze upon a doubtful work of art. By degrees, a horrible remembrance of one branch of her calling took possession of the woman; and stooping down, she pinned his wandering arms against his sides, to see how he would look if laid out as a dead man. Her fingers itched to compose his limbs in that last marble attitude. "Ah!" said Mrs Gamp, walking away from the bed, "he'd make a lovely corpse."
>
> She now proceeded to unpack her bundle; lighted a candle with the aid of a fire-box on the drawers; filled a small kettle, as a preliminary to refreshing herself with a cup of tea in the course of the night; laid what she called "a little bit of fire," for the same philanthropic purpose; and also set forth a small tea-board, that nothing might be wanting for her comfortable enjoyment. These preparations occupied so long, that when they were brought to a conclusion it was high time to think about supper; so she rang the bell and ordered it.

Once Mrs Gamp has finished her supper she sits back in her chair and reflects:

> "What a blessed thing it is to make sick people happy in their beds, and never mind one's self as long as one can do a service!"
>
> She moralised in the same vein until her glass was empty, and then administered the patient's medicine, by the simple process of clutching his windpipe to make him gasp, and immediately pouring it down his throat. "I a'most forgot the piller, I declare!" said Mrs Gamp, drawing it away. "There! Now he's comfortable as he can be, I'm sure! I must try to make myself as much so as I can."
>
> With this view, she went about the construction of an extemporaneous bed in the easy-chair, with the addition of the next easy one for her feet.

The next morning Mrs Gamp reports to the doctor and greets her colleague.

> "Well!" said the doctor, "we must keep him quiet; keep the room cool; give him his draughts regularly; and see that he's carefully looked to. That's all!"
>
> "And as long as Mrs Prig and me waits upon him, sir, no fear of that," said Mrs Gamp.
>
> "I suppose," observed Mrs Prig, when they had curtseyed the doctor out, "there's nothin' new?"
>
> "Nothin' at all, my dear," said Mrs Gamp. "He's rather wearin' in his talk from making up a lot of names; elseways you needn't mind him."
>
> "Oh, I shan't mind him," Mrs Prig returned. "I have somethin' else to think of."

6. Some Reflections on Mrs Gamp

Not every reader will find the exploits of Mrs Gamp amusing, although in my experience most people cannot help but laugh at the extract. However, I believe that the irony of the piece, amusing or not, is obvious. The interesting question, however, is *why* such a piece of prose works as irony? Without straying too far into the realm of literary criticism, I believe we can give a reasonable account of the ironic effect in terms of the juxtaposition of the world as revealed in the text against our own experiences and expectations. The text clashes with our moral sensibilities; and this is emphatically not a clash merely in taste. The irony works because there is a justified presumption concerning the right moral starting point in such caring relationships as that between healthcare worker and patient.

It may well be true that when Dickens conceived of the character he was relying for his caricature upon the real social phenomenon of the so-called "nurse" of disreputable character, whose role was yet to be superseded by the development of professional nursing. However, the irony evident in the account of Mrs Gamp's behavior works now, and I would suggest worked then, because we already know, or at least have expectations about, what ought to follow in terms of behavior when a person has a duty of care towards another.

But what is the right moral starting point for such behavior? We can go some way to establishing the parameters here if we consider the Mrs Gamp example in a different context. Imagine for example that you are a tutor responsible for educating novice healthcare workers and that Mrs Gamp is a candidate student for your education and training program. It seems to me that we can begin with some quite concrete ideas about what we would need Mrs Gamp to grasp in order for her to progress as a student, and here I am implying that part of the assessment of progress for a student healthcare worker necessarily includes an evaluation of the student's personal moral progress. I do not mean to suggest that novice healthcare workers enter the profession as moral deviants and are somehow converted into paragons of virtue by the training program. Rather, I am suggesting that it is the business of such programs to attend to ethics education not only with a view about where, in terms of moral development, the student ought to be at the end of the program, but with a clear idea of what the premises for such a program ought to be. With reference to my earlier reflections on teleology, such programs usually do have a teleological schema well worked out in terms of the aims and objectives of the program, or in terms of the behavioral criteria the student must demonstrate in order to be judged competent.

Mrs Gamp is of course a convenient device, an obvious if crude caricature, through which to make explicit the parameters involved in facilitating personal moral progress; however, noting this fact does not detract from the validity of the example. The following schema captures at least some of the parameters on which the progress of a student on such a program of education might be based.

- Mapping the moral domain—acquainting the person with the givens.
- Developing a sense of moral relevance.
- Self-scrutiny or moral reflection—challenging shallow understanding of moral concepts.

Using Mrs Gamp as the subject, I shall now give some substance to the three specimen categories identified in the above schema.

A. Mapping the Moral Domain

Mrs Gamp is clearly an extreme case, in need of quite remedial moral education, as witnessed by the example of her caring endeavors. We would hope that Mrs Gamp is not a typical example of the average novice healthcare worker. However, mapping the moral domain with any healthcare workers requires the establishment of some clear parameters or "givens." Understanding and assimilating such givens would constitute personal progress for the student. Of course, the givens may also constitute the point of departure for still further progress, although this raises possibilities that I do not wish to consider here. I will, however, say something on this issue below.

Progress construed in terms of "outcomes" for the student could be identified as, for example, observable behaviors in the student as she enters the sickroom. For example, we would expect the healthcare worker to have a certain orientation, demonstrate a particular phenomenological perspective, which shows her to perceive the very room as having a certain kind of moral salience. The focus of the healthcare worker's attention ought to be directed toward the person who is the patient. The objects in the room ought to be regarded as means to serve the interests of the patient and not, as Mrs Gamp regards the room and its contents, as potential vehicles for her personal comfort. The irony of the exchange between Mrs Prig and Mrs Gamp, for example, is that it inverts the expected priorities, focusing as it does on the quality of the food and amenities for the carer rather than for the patient. Others have commented upon this sense of moral salience when describing the relationship between health worker and patient. Søren Holm states:

> When you meet the patient you meet another human being who is vulnerable, who trusts you, and whose life you can influence in a significant way. This creates a specific responsibility towards this human being, which can be difficult to understand for outsiders, but which nevertheless plays a significant role in the deliberation of health care professionals. In their minds it is related to the power they have, and to the respect they have to show.[9]

Nurse theorists have described this relationship as one imbued with care.[10] However it is characterized, the relationship between healthcare worker and patient ought to be a moral relationship which stands out as different to that between strangers meeting on the street, or that between customer and sales assistant. To understand the moral nature of the relationship is to understand the implicit set of priorities that form the parameters of adopting such a role: for example, that there may be some sacrifice of personal comfort or preferences by the healthcare worker in favor of the comfort and preferences of the patient. These are at least the starting premises of such a relationship.

B. Developing a Sense of Moral Relevance

Developing a sense of moral relevance would seem to follow on from a basic mapping of the moral domain. An understanding of such diverse moral concepts as duty, compassion, obligation, and trust would seem to stem from a fundamental grasp of the distinction between the self and the other, and the multitude of possible relationships, with their implied priorities, which are possible between one person and another. Perhaps Mrs Gamp believes that she has fulfilled her duty by sitting with her patient all night and ensuring that he received his medication. This, I would suggest, is because she is not able to distinguish between the merely functional care of "care-taking" and "taking care"—what Per Nortvedt describes as "being-for-the-other."[11]

We might begin to be convinced that Mrs Gamp had indeed made progress if we witnessed her ability to recognize the difference between cared and cared for, and saw her incorporating such differences, in a variety of ways, into her routine of care. The development of a disposition or habit of care would demonstrate a deepening of Mrs Gamp's moral understanding, and such changes in behavior would be evidence of her personal moral progress.

C. Self-Scrutiny or Capacity for Moral Reflection

Closely tied to this deepening moral sense and evolving disposition to act in a morally appropriate way towards her patients, would be evidence of an evolving capacity for reflexivity. By reflexivity, I mean the capacity to engage in a process of reflection, making oneself aware of the processes involved in making a judgment and turning such judgment into action with the purpose of reinforcing or revising those processes. This is a critical capacity, which the student might be required, and ought to be able, to make explicit in an accessible way.

In my account of personal moral progress through a model of professional education, I have tried to give a flavor rather than a detailed account of what the process might consist in. It is clearly not a comprehensive account. However, I believe that we would judge our student, Mrs Gamp, to have undergone a process of personal moral development, if at the end of the period of education she was able to demonstrate, both in how she justified her actions and in how she consistently behaved, that she had assimilated the values upon which healthcare is premised. There are of course some outstanding questions. How can we be sure of the validity of the preconceptions that formed the premises of the educators? How can we be sure that the goals to which students have to progress, are themselves "progressed" positions? As with other areas of knowledge, it is more reasonable to presume against the skeptic than with her.[12]

Some questions are no longer open. The question of whether a patient is deserving of respect, sympathy, and care is not something that has to be established anew with each case. If this claim is not convincing, then try the Dickens test, since nothing, I am sure, could change our minds so completely as to enable us to read the passages from Dickens as purely descriptive with not a shred of irony about them. Even less could we be convinced that this was a textbook example of good nursing care. This is not to say that the premises of healthcare ethics are not themselves open to revision. Of course they are, and so ought they to be. Naked paternalism has been rightly challenged as the single foundation for the relationship between health worker and patient. But the understanding of the concept of autonomy that helped to oust paternalism is undergoing a further transition, as we attempt to enrich it and render it more subtle, more sensitive to the complex situations in which healthcare is practiced.

The idea that we have gained moral knowledge, that we do presume to have established some moral baselines as our starting point, are the sorts of point I believe hold not only for my example of personal moral progress, but more generally. Godlovitch characterizes such progress as "ratcheting-up."[13] A ratchet is a mechanism incorporated into some tools to prevent any backwards slippage, and thus technology provides a useful model for a test of moral progress: the "slippage test." On this basis he argues that we could no more revert to an internalized acceptance of racial superiority or sexism than we could to a pre-Copernican cosmology. Put this way, some such developments in moral thinking do seem nigh-on irreversible, and establish what might be called—in a term that would be anathema to post-modernists—central tenets of morality.

NOTES

1. Keith Michael Baker, *Condorcet: From Natural Philosophy to Social Mathematics* (Chicago, IL: University of Chicago Press, 1975), p. 350.

2. Charles Taylor, *Sources of the Self* (Cambridge: Cambridge University Press), p. 63.

3. Michele Moody-Adams, "The Idea of Moral Progress," *Metaphilosophy*, 30:3 (July 1999), pp. 168–185.

4. Thomas Nagel, *The View From Nowhere* (New York, NY: Oxford University Press, 1986).

5. Peter Singer, *Rethinking Life and Death* (New York, NY: Oxford University Press, 1994).

6. Taylor, *Sources of the Self*, p. 72.

7. Stan Godlovitch, "Morally We Roll Along: (Optimistic Reflections) on Moral Progress," *Journal of Applied Philosophy,* 15:3 (1998), pp. 271–286.

8. Charles Dickens, *Martin Chuzzlewit* (Oxford: Oxford University Press, 1998), pp. 345–358.

9. Søren Holm, *Ethical Problems in Clinical Practice* (Manchester: Manchester University Press, 1997), p. 127.

10. P. Anne Scott, "Emotion, Moral Perception, and Nursing," *Nursing Philosophy*, 1:2 (October 2000), pp. 123–133.

11. Per Nortvedt, "Sensitive Judgement: An Enquiry into the Foundations of Nursing Ethics," *Nursing Ethics*, 5:5 (September 1998), p. 385.

12. Ronald Dworkin, "Objectivity and Truth: You'd Better Believe it," *Philosophy and Public Affairs*, 25:2 (Spring 1996), pp. 87–139.

13. Godlovitch, "Morally We Roll Along."

Thirteen

HEALTHCARE AND
(A KIND OF) VIRTUE ETHICS

Mark Sheehan

1. "Non-Normative" Virtue Bioethics

My aim here is to sketch the beginnings of what I take to be a distinctive approach to bioethics. It is an approach that arises from the application of a particular position in metaethics to ethical issues in medicine and healthcare. In what follows I will give a (very) brief account of the position, trying to highlight the most salient aspects for its application. In the second part of the chapter I will consider how in general terms this approach to metaethics might be effectively applied to the realm of medicine and healthcare. As I hope we will see, it results in a kind of virtue bioethics.

One way of saying what is distinctive about virtue theory is by reference to the question that is taken as the starting point of ethical reflection. Virtue theory, as I will understand it, has as its focus the question "What kind of person should I be?" as opposed to the question "What ought I to do?" What makes the approach that I want to suggest here a virtue ethics approach is not much more than its connection with the former rather than the latter question.

Starting with, as it were, an agent-based question (What kind of person should I be?) rather than the act-based question (What ought I to do?) can lead the theorist in one of two ways. First, by analyzing the virtuous person's character, we might be able to elicit some helpful insights into what ought to be done in certain kinds of situations. This would begin to give content to the claim that the right thing to do in a situation is what the virtuous person would do in that situation. If we can develop some idea of what characteristics the virtuous person possesses (that is, the virtues) then, the thought goes, we will have a better idea of what ought to be done. The idea is that by focusing on the first question, we will be better placed to answer the second.

Alternatively, we might think that beginning with the agent-based question leads us away from an answer to the act-based question. That is, once we have decided that the right thing to do in a given situation is what the virtuous person would do in that situation, there is not much more to be said that will enable us to determine what ought to be done. Taking this second route leads us to focus on what it is that the virtuous person can do—what abilities and capacities does the virtuous person possess that facilitates right moral judgment? Importantly, this question is not concerned with which judgments are right, but with what enables one to make judgments that are right. It is this second route that I will take in this chapter.

It might reasonably be expected that a virtue theory would make some mention of the nature or content of the virtues, but I will not—so, it is only "a kind of" virtue theory. The reason for this is partly to distinguish the account from normative virtue ethics—the first path above. Normative virtue ethics, like all normative theories, in the end, tells us what we ought to do. My approach here is a metaethical one, and so it does not attempt to do this—at least for the most part. Instead it makes claims about, among other things, the nature of ethics, and more specifically about the particular capacity possessed by the virtuous agent. I say "for the most part" here because there will be some substantive normative claims that the approach will generate, but its primary aim is not to generate such claims, nor is its aim to provide a systematic set of formulae for their generation.

2. Metaethics

The theoretical position I will discuss here traces its roots, like most "virtue-style" approaches, to Aristotle's *Nicomachean Ethics*. On one reading of Aristotle he has very little to say in the *Nicomachean Ethics* that has normative content. Indeed, as David Wiggins has put it, "everything hard has been permitted to take refuge in the notion of *aisthesis*, or situational appreciation … And in *aisthesis*, as Aristotle says, explanations give out."[1] So while Aristotle does spend some time dealing with character and with the nature of the virtues, in the end the exercise of virtue depends on practical reason and judgment: "[T]he temperate man craves for the things he ought, as he ought, and when he ought; and this is what rational principle directs."[2]

There are two aspects of this theoretical position that I want to bring out here. The first is the kind of perceptual capacity or "situational appreciation" that is possessed by the virtuous agent. John McDowell suggests that:

> A kind person can be relied on to behave kindly when that is what the situation requires. Moreover, his reliably kind behaviour is not the outcome of a blind, non-rational habit or instinct … Rather, that the situation requires a certain sort of behaviour is (one way of formulating) his reason for behaving in that way, on each of the relevant occasions. So it must be something of which, on each of the relevant occasions, he is aware. A kind person has a reliable sensitivity to a certain sort of requirement that situations impose on behaviour. The deliverances of a reliable sensitivity are cases of knowledge …The sensitivity is, we might say, a sort of perceptual capacity.[3]

This perceptual capacity is the core of the approach. It is this special sensitivity, aided and influenced by reflection and deliberation, that enables the virtuous agent to recognize and respond to the requirements of particular contexts.

The second aspect of the position that should be mentioned here involves the justification of particular moral judgments. McDowell suggests that:

> In urging behaviour one takes to be morally required, one finds oneself saying things like this: "You don't know what it means that someone is shy and sensitive." Conveying what a circumstance means, in this loaded sense, is getting someone to see it in the special way in which a virtuous person would see it. In the attempt to do so, one exploits contrivances similar to those one exploits in other areas where the task is to back up the injunction "See it like this": helpful juxtapositions of cases, descriptions with carefully chosen terms and carefully placed emphasis, and the like.[4]

In the attempt to get a person to see matters aright—to argue for, defend, or justify a particular claim—one exploits a variety of contrivances. This variety is not to be underestimated. It includes consequence-based and deontic considerations, logic, emotion, character, and, for want of a better term, conceptual analysis. In short, it includes the full gamut of argumentative strategies and the complex conceptual apparatus provided by ordinary language.

So, the key thought behind this approach is that the virtuous person has a special perceptual ability. This enables our virtuous person to recognize, read, or interpret situations well. The recognizing, reading, and so on, amount to determining what ought to be done in those situations. But of course this says nothing of the kind of justification that can be used to support the deliverances of this sensitivity. In normative ethics, moral theorists of particular persuasions each have their own justificatory strategies. So, for example, the utilitarian might justify her judgments by reference to the utilitarian calculus of expected utility. With this approach (and this is related to it being a metaethical approach), there is no one justificatory strategy—there is no definitive set of rules to follow or no calculus to employ. Instead, all considerations and all justificatory strategies are available and, before the fact, equally relevant. Again, in the end the judgment about which justificatory strategy is conclusive in a particular case depends on the case and on the ability of the judge to see what is to be done.

I want now to mention two of the more standard objections to this approach, if only to put them aside. First, we might be concerned about relativism and moral truth. How is this even vaguely a realist position? How can there be a "fact of the matter" about what ought to be done if there is no fixed justificatory strategy for assessing truth, and judgments of obligation rest or depend upon the agent's "perception?" This is, I think, the most difficult problem faced by this account and so, naturally, it is one that I am not going to deal with here. Some work has been done on it, and much needs to be done. By and large this view does accept a reasonable amount of relativism at the level of the particular judgments made by agents. It does however hold that these judgments "aspire to truth," as David Wiggins has put it, and that in some cases this is achieved.[5]

Second, it might be complained that we really want our moral theory to tell us what ought to be done—"At least normative virtue ethics does that!"—but this metaethical approach shies away from providing anything that is of use. The response here is to make an "anti-normative theory" point: that searching for the one, true normative theory is a mistaken enterprise and should, in the face of the way in which our moral lives go, be given up. This claim depends on the distinctiveness of particular contexts and the inadequacy of rules and principles to cover this distinctiveness—that is, independently of a particular sensitivity concerning their application. As McDowell puts it:

> If one attempted to reduce one's conception of what virtue requires to a set of rules, then, however subtle and thoughtful one was in drawing up the code, cases would inevitably turn up in which a mechanical application of the rules would strike one as wrong—and not necessarily because one had changed one's mind; rather, one's mind on the matter was not susceptible of capture in any universal formula.[6]

This is not to say that rules, generalizations, outcomes, evidence, and the like play no role or are of no consequence. They feature only as appropriate and only as called for by the situation itself.

3. Applications to Medicine and Healthcare

As things stand one would be justified in thinking that this theoretical approach could provide very little in the way of assistance to those concerned with ethical issues in healthcare. Indeed, the interesting ethical issues that arise in healthcare are all normative ones—those about which this approach is silent. How then, could an approach such as this provide anything satisfactory in the realm of healthcare? The answer comes in two parts: first, in practical terms, by developing and encouraging what we might broadly call "moral seriousness," and second (more theoretically) by a more thorough examination of the idea of a "practice" as it applies to the practice of medicine. Each of these will be discussed briefly below.

First, this approach, given its Aristotelian roots, places a significant emphasis on education, reflection, and experience. This of course ties to the "perception-sensitivity" points—we develop the perceptual capacity in question precisely through some combination of these. It is the agent, in context, who is to decide what ought to be done, and the agent who must be sensitive to the nuances of the situation. Education, reflection, and experience prepare the agent for such decision-making and each requires, in the end, that the agent take seriously the business of ethics. As Aristotle points out, the "youthful in character" are not the proper hearers of his lectures:

> For to such persons, as to the incontinent, knowledge brings no profit; but to those who desire and act in accordance with a rational principle knowledge about such matters will be of great benefit.[7]

It might be thought, however, that this appeal to Aristotelian aspirations or "moral seriousness" is merely a toothless platitude—"Everyone knows that education, reflection, and experience are important. No sane ethicist would deny it." But if this is the *limit*, if education, reflection, and experience are all that ethics and ethicists can provide, this begins to bite quite deeply. Many, perhaps most, members of the healthcare community are used to the methodology of science. Science provides definitive answers to problems. The same is often expected of ethics. On this account though, the nature of ethics is such that the kind of guidance often expected—definitive rules or algorithms that will yield solutions—cannot be provided. There is a good deal more to be said on these matters. However, the main point to stress here is that this approach does have significant consequences for healthcare and, in particular, for the relationship between healthcare and ethics. Ethics (as a discipline) provides a distinctive kind of practical education about the patterns and forms of moral argumentation and justification.

A second way in which the theoretical position outlined in the last section can be applied to healthcare is by exploring the idea of "a practice," and utilizing it in the case of the practice of medicine. The main connection between virtue theory and the idea of a practice as a theoretical term comes from the work of Alasdair MacIntyre and, in particular, his *After Virtue*. There he defines a practice as:

> any coherent and complex form of socially established cooperative human activity through which goods internal to that form of activity are realized in the course of trying to achieve those standards of excellence which are appropriate to, and partially derivative of, that form of activity, with the result that human powers to achieve excellence, and human conceptions of the ends and goods involved, are systematically extended.[8]

So, bricklaying is not a practice but architecture is. Kicking a football skilfully is not a practice but the game of football is. Planting turnips is not a practice but farming is.

Much of this definition is not particularly relevant to the discussion here, concerned as it is with MacIntyre's general theoretical position and the linkages between practices, narratives, and the unity of a tradition. Very briefly, MacIntyre's account of virtues

> proceeds through three stages: a first which considers virtues as qualities necessary to achieve the goods internal to practices; a second which considers them as qualities contributing to a whole life; and a third which relates them to the pursuit of a good for human beings the conception of which can only be elaborated and possessed within an ongoing social tradition.[9]

In all of this, "no human quality is to be accounted a virtue unless it satisfies the conditions specified *at each of the three stages*."[10]

To further explain his idea of a practice MacIntyre uses, among others, the example of the practice of playing chess. If we wanted to teach an unwilling child to play chess we might initially require some external incentive (candy), but we would hope that there will

> come a time when the child will find in those goods specific to chess, in the achievement of a certain highly particular kind of analytical skill, strategic imagination, and competitive intensity, a new set of reasons … for trying to excel in whatever way the game of chess requires.[11]

MacIntyre is not as clear as he might be about the relationship between goods internal to a practice and the practice itself. It is perhaps safest to define the relation negatively, in terms of external goods:

> There are always alternative ways of achieving (external) goods, and their achievement is never to be had *only* by engaging in some particular kind of practice.[12]

There is a little more to the connection between the idea of a practice and virtue theory than the MacIntyrean one. Virtue theories tend to be teleological. That is, the virtues, it is normally held, are characteristics required for the Good Life, where the Good Life is to be understood as the goal, or end, or point of human life. Given this, it should be reasonably clear why "practices" are useful units of analysis for virtue theorists like MacIntyre. Practices, characterized in part by the goods internal to each of them, can readily be seen as component parts of human life. Each of these component parts can, with varying degrees of ease, be separated out from the rest and examined. Of course, the rest of MacIntyre's structure is designed to capture the way in which the vast array of practices in which an individual might participate are to be combined to make sense of a life in a particular society. In any case, for our purposes here the unit of the practice provides us with a smaller, more limited group of human interactions. This hopefully makes the specification and investigation of normative requirements more manageable. The link with teleology is also of use here. First, although we might be skeptical about the possibility of saying much about the *telos* of human life, this might not be as much of a problem for particular practices. Second, the goal or point of a practice is an additional tool with which to understand normative requirements. This is, I think, true at both the normative and metaethical levels. By reflecting on the practice of medicine and her place in it, the individual has an additional justificatory tool to use in the process of decision-making. But also, it will I think turn out in this case that the point of the practice of medicine and what gives it its sense will provide us with internal grounds for the obligations of those who participate in it.

When we do turn to the application of this idea to healthcare we are immediately confronted by a problem of scope. What exactly is the relevant practice? Healthcare might be taken to be not one but many different practices. Alternatively, it seems perhaps extreme to distinguish the practices within healthcare too finely—by distinguishing, say, the practice of obstetrics from the practice of gynecology. Certainly, in a fully worked out account these issues would need to be addressed, but in the context of this chapter it is not unreasonable to allow a degree of abstraction. With this in mind, I will primarily be concerned in what follows with clinical medicine and, consequently, with the practice of clinical medicine. Physicians wear many hats. I will not be considering the physician as scientist or the physician as citizen. The ethical issues that arise in the context of research are distinct from those in clinical medicine. Similarly, while the social and political issues involved in medicine very often impinge on clinical medicine, the ethical issues surrounding rationing and distributive justice (for instance) are also distinct. This is not meant to imply that there is no overlap or that the distinctions are always and everywhere clear. Clinical medicine is, I think, quite readily seen as a practice in MacIntyre's sense, and it is one that perhaps unjustly (given the variety of healthcare provision) receives much attention (consider here discussions of the physician-patient relationship).

It is important to be a little clearer about the relationship between these considerations concerning the idea of a practice and the metaethical position of the previous section. If this account of a practice and its application are used to inform the individual's understanding of his or her obligations or values then, naturally, the strategy is being used as a method of justification or reasoning. Given my metaethical position, the use of this strategy as a form of moral reasoning stands on an equal footing with any other form of reasoning. That is, my claim is not that the normative results that follow from using this method to determine one's obligations are to be privileged over any other method. In this respect, my brief discussion of the practice of medicine below is not intended to violate the non-normative requirement of the metaethical position of the first section. So, the thought is that once we have given an account of the practice of medicine, we have not necessarily exhausted the ethical considerations. We might, for instance, still ask whether this practice and its internal goods are themselves the sorts of things that we should have in our society or, more generally, whether this practice coheres with other values and practices.

4. Internal Morality and the Practice of Medicine

These general thoughts about applying a virtue theoretic approach to medicine and healthcare have recently received some attention. A 2001 issue of the *Journal of Medicine and Philosophy* was dedicated to what is known as the "internal morality of medicine." Central to the idea of an internal morality of medicine is the MacIntyrean account of a practice and of the goods internal to a practice.[13] The internal morality step is obtained in the case of medicine because, it is thought, medicine constitutes a practice and so has internal goods. These internal goods provide us with the tools for an internal morality of medicine: a morality, for healthcare professionals, built around the internal goods of the practice. In this last section, I will briefly look at the way in which this discussion utilizes and so applies MacIntyre's idea of a practice to medicine and healthcare. We will see that in so applying the idea of a practice there are a number of temptations that we would do well to avoid. The chapter will conclude with a few general remarks about the practice of medicine and the way in which this "kind of" virtue ethics might proceed.

A. Mistaken Views of "Practice"

Perhaps the most significant danger in applying the idea of a practice to any particular case is that we focus too heavily on the goods internal to that practice. Edmund Pellegrino, in his paper on the internal morality of medicine is I think guilty of this, as are Robert Veatch and Tom Beauchamp.[14] Pellegrino writes that the practice of medicine

> exists because being ill and being healed are universal human experiences, not because society has created medicine as a practice. Rather than social construct, the nature of medicine, its internal goods and virtues, are defined by the ends of medicine itself, and therefore, ontologically internal from the outset.[15]

So it looks as though the goods of medicine come from the nature of medicine, and that the goods internal to the practice of medicine are the same as the goods or ends of medicine.

There are two general dangers that this account highlights. First, we should be careful not to assume that the relationship between the practice of medicine and the nature of medicine is clear. The nature of medicine might very well be fixed but the form of the activity, the practice, might vary. Pellegrino seems to miss the fact that practices, in MacIntyre's sense, are intrinsically social and so must be social constructions in an important sense. Of course this is not to deny that there might be constraining facts of the matter that limit and shape this construction. But it is to be expected that different people, in different cultures and in different circumstances, will appropriate medicine differently. The underlying concern in all of this is that the goods and goals of the "science of medicine" are being too closely linked with the goods internal to the practice of medicine.

The second danger involved in applying MacIntyre's account of a practice to medicine is that we will focus too hard on the *goods* internal to the practice, and not on other normative features internal to it. It is interesting to note, in this context, that MacIntyre's definition of a practice refers to the standards of excellence appropriate to particular practices in addition to the goods internal to them. It is also easy to miss the ordinariness in MacIntyre's definition of a practice—the fact that a practice is a complex activity or set of activities that involves particular kinds of relationships in very particular sets of circumstances. Indeed, a good case can be made for thinking that the physician-patient relationship is of a unique sort. It would not be surprising, then, if there were unique obligations and responsibilities that attached to both sides of it.

B. Internal Morality and the Practice of Medicine

There is one final danger associated with using the idea of a practice to explicate morality within medicine. This danger involves another way of failing to distinguish between various senses of the practice of medicine. While it does apply in cases like Pellegrino's account, it is only in the background, and as I have suggested, there are more pressing concerns in his case.

A useful way to bring this danger out is with reference to Plato's *Republic*. In Book One, Socrates uses the physician as an example in his discussion with Thrasymachus regarding the nature of justice. In the example, he considers the science of medicine to be an art, and the physician to be the stronger and the patient to be the weaker. He also distinguishes between the strict and the popular senses of a word. Thus the physician in the strict sense is not someone who can be mistaken about medicine, nor is the physician in the strict sense one who makes money or earns fees. Socrates claims that "any physician in so far as he is a physician seek(s) or enjoin(s) the advantage ... of the patient."[16] The methodology in this part of the text and, arguably, the point of the discussion as a whole is that, by considering and understanding what it is to be a physician in the strict sense, we shall come to see that the "true" physician seeks the advantage of the patient. That is, by investigating what it means to be a physician in the strict sense, we might become clearer about the way in which a physician ought to behave.

Clearly we are not concerned with the argument of the Republic or with Platonic bioethics. Indeed, really, the use of medicine as an example is not important to the point at hand. What is most important here is the distinction between the physician and the physician in the strict sense. One way of cashing out this distinction is to distinguish between actual physicians and the concept of a physician. (I do not mean to imply that this is how Socrates intended the distinction to be drawn, though I think that there is a plausible reading of Book One that draws the distinction in something like this way.) So the physician in the strict sense cannot be mistaken, does not earn money, and seeks the advantage of the patient. It is very important to distinguish between the concept of a physician and the ideal physician. Very roughly and for our purposes here, the former is tied to meaning and language in a way that the latter is not.

In the context of the practice of medicine, it is the "strict sense" of the practice with which we are concerned. The final danger to be wary of in investigating the practice of medicine then, is failing to distinguish this strict sense of the practice of medicine from the practice of medicine in actual contexts on the one hand, and some notion of the ideal practice of medicine on the other. To a large extent, the difference between each of these involves a difference in methodological approach. If we wished to study the actual practice of medicine we would conduct an empirical study. An investigation into the ideal practice of medicine, naturally, takes us directly into first order normative ethical theory—presumably detailing how physicians ought to act involves giving substance to a conception of the ideal practice.

Since our focus is on something more like the concept of the practice of medicine, our investigation would utilize the resources of conceptual analysis. In such a study, the relationship between the facts about the practice in a particular context—the way medicine is practiced—and the concept of "the practice of medicine" is importantly normative. A complete account of the concept will enable us to criticize particular instances of the practice in various ways, and it will contribute to accounts of the ideal practice in an important way. Much more needs to be said about these methodologies and, in particular, about the one favored here—however this requires a separate project. It is important to notice how this approach links with the metaethical approach described above. This "linguistic strategy" is not one that is available only to this approach, but is essentially a metaethical strategy and so is particularly germane to a metaethical approach.

The Socratic example of medicine involved a three-way relationship between the science of medicine, the physician, and the patient. We might roughly understand the science of medicine to involve, particularly, the body of knowledge, given by science, concerning the human body. Thus, the physician is ideally someone who possesses this knowledge and has the skill to apply it. The patient, by and large, does not possess either this knowledge or the skill to apply it, and yet she has needs or deficiencies that she thinks can be met or remedied. The practice of medicine will then be the cooperative activity of applying this knowledge and skill, in the context of the relationships that must be formed in the process. The forms that the relationships involved in this activity take will be largely determined by two features: the expectations and motivations that those entering the practice have, and the limits and relevance of the body of knowledge to the goals informing those motivations and expectations. It seems clear that patients are motivated to visit physicians by what they understand to be their needs and the relevance of the physician's skill to those needs. They might expect, given this, that the physician will endeavour to meet those needs. It is fair to say, also, that physicians can expect that patients will have these motivations and expectations about their needs and the physician's relation to them. Of course the relationship generally is affected by the disparity of knowledge between the physician and the patient. Quite clearly, even with the recent advances in medicine, there will be things that cannot be achieved by the physician (or by any physician). Similarly, there will be some matters about which medicine will have nothing to say.

The idea is that by giving an account of the practice of medicine, understood broadly as I have suggested above, we can isolate certain kinds of relationships and goals that are constitutive of, or at least intimately involved in, the practice. These relationships are formed between people who have general kinds of expectations, motivations, and goals. So, what it means to be a physician in the strict sense—understood as an essential component of the practice—is tied to the practice and its point. This, in turn, is understood in terms of the relationships and goals that are constitutive of the practice. This kind of approach avoids the difficulties that beset other attempts to apply the idea of a practice to healthcare. It does not assume that a practice is defined or constituted by the goods internal to it. The resulting account would not involve recourse to external normative principles or normative theory, and in this sense it would be an internal bioethics. It would of course be intimately related to the metaethical position informing it, and in this sense it would be a kind of virtue bioethics.

NOTES

1. David Wiggins, "Deliberation and Practical Reason," *Needs, Values, Truth*, ed. David Wiggins (Oxford: Clarendon Press, 3rd ed.,1998), p. 237.

2. Aristotle, *Nicomachean Ethics*, trans. David Ross, revised by J. O. Urmson and J. L. Ackrill (Oxford: Oxford University Press, 1998), 1119b15–19.

3. John McDowell, *Mind, Value, and Reality* (London: Harvard University Press, 1998) p. 51.

4. McDowell, *Mind, Value, and Reality*, p. 85.

5. David Wiggins, "Moral Cognitivism, Moral Relativism, and Motivating Moral Beliefs," *Proceedings of the Aristotelian Society*, 91 (1990), pp. 61–85.

6. McDowell, *Mind, Value, and Reality*, p. 58.

7. Aristotle, *Nicomachean Ethics*, 1095a9–12.

8. Alasdair MacIntyre, *After Virtue* (London: Duckworth, 3rd ed., 1985), p. 187.

9. *Ibid*., p. 273.

10. *Ibid*., p. 275.

11. *Ibid*., p. 187.

12. *Ibid*., p. 187.

13. Robert M. Veatch and Franklin G. Miller, "The Internal Morality of Medicine: An Introduction," *Journal of Medicine and Philosophy*, 26:6 (2001), pp. 555–556.

14. Robert M. Veatch, "The Impossibility of a Morality Internal to Medicine," *Journal of Medicine and Philosophy*, 26:6 (2001), pp. 621–642; Tom L. Beauchamp, "Internal and External Standards for Medical Morality," *Journal of Medicine and Philosophy*, 26:6 (2001), pp. 601–619.

15. Edmund D. Pellegrino, "The Internal Morality of Clinical Medicine: A Paradigm for the Ethics of the Helping and Healing Professions," *Journal of Medicine and Philosophy*, 26:6 (2001), p. 563.

16. Plato, *The Republic*, trans. Robin Waterfield (Oxford: Oxford University Press, 1998), 342d3–6.

Fourteen

BIOETHICS, RIGHTS-BASED CONSEQUENTIALISM, AND SOCIAL REALITY

Peter Herissone-Kelly

1. Four Aims

I have four aims in this chapter. First, I want to sketch a possible non-utilitarian rights-based consequentialist approach to philosophical bioethics, an approach that attempts to give rights their proper place in moral theory by attributing to them an independent, non-derivative value. Second, I want to examine an objection to such an approach, an objection that says that rights can never be properly accommodated within a consequentialist framework. The thought that I will develop here is that consequentialism, no matter how much we tinker with it, can never be harmonized with the view of persons upon which the notion of a right depends, and so will always "miss the point" of rights. Third, I will suggest that perhaps this objection, sound though it may be, is of little relevance to many of the issues dealt with in bioethics. This is because consequentialist and non-consequentialist approaches to rights appear to collapse into each other when applied to the sorts of questions of policy with which much of bioethics deals. Finally, I will point out how unsatisfactory, and how much of a puzzle, this is: it appears that the way of thinking of persons that underlies the attribution to them of rights tends of necessity to disappear precisely when we most need it.

The first two aims will involve a fairly substantial detour into some general moral theory, while the third and fourth will bring me firmly back into the realm of bioethics. The detour is necessary if we are to end up at the correct destination.

2. Consequentialism and Rights

Imagine a callow young philosopher eager to develop a research interest in bioethics. She is convinced, rightly or wrongly (though surely not unfeasibly), that bioethics requires moral theory, and she finds that she has strong consequentialist intuitions. She recognizes that her most natural choice of theory—and here, she would certainly have lots of company amongst bioethicists—is utilitarianism, but something worries her about the doctrine.

It displays an irritating tendency to clash with another set of intuitions that she holds. That is, there are concepts that seem indispensable to a proper understanding of bioethical issues that utilitarianism just does not seem able to accommodate, or at least not in quite the right way. Chief amongst these concepts is that of a right.

Of course, she is aware that a utilitarianism of any sophistication is more than ready to offer utilitarian justifications of the notion of rights. And it is worth noting that all versions of utilitarianism bar the caricature of that theory presented to first year undergraduates *are* sophisticated. But still her unease remains.

Her disquiet might be explained in the following way. Utilitarian justifications of rights necessarily afford them a subordinate, derivative value, a value dependent on their contribution to general happiness or, in modern varieties of utilitarianism, preference satisfaction. And our bioethicist's intuition might be that this is just not good enough—that rights have an independent, non-derivative value.

The utilitarian may attempt to counter the fledgling bioethicist's worries by asking what difference it makes to believe this, so long as the utilitarian calculations deliver the answer she desires: so long, that is, as rights end up being respected. But quite apart from the fact that she might just want to get clear about what sorts of value (derivative or non-derivative) the various elements of her moral theory have, this suggestion is unlikely to appear very soothing. If she genuinely thinks—again, despite all her consequentialist leanings—that rights have a non-derivative value, then a utilitarianism that makes them subordinate to preference satisfaction will inevitably present the appearance of a rogue theory. That is, it might as a matter of fact invariably recommend actions that respect rights, but there always remains the possibility that it will throw up what from her perspective is the wrong answer. Rights could be trampled on at any moment, if such trampling turns out to maximize preference satisfaction.

What is the bioethicist do in this imagined situation? Her intuitions are robustly consequentialist, but she also has a commitment to the non-derivative status of rights, and that commitment is usually thought of as deontological in character. The alternative, it seems to me, is for her to adopt a non-utilitarian consequentialism that confers an independent, *sui generis* value on rights. Of course, many would call this a variety of ideal utilitarianism (a utilitarianism that admits a plurality of independent values into its axiology, or theory of the good). Anne Maclean would call it an impure utilitarianism.[1] While I think it more useful to call it rights-based consequentialism, and to reserve the term "utilitarianism" for that variety of consequentialism that posits either happiness or preference satisfaction as the sole independent good, I am ultimately unconcerned with nomenclature. What I am concerned to do is to outline, and look at the prospects for, a consequentialism that is prepared to regard rights as possessed of a non-derivative value.

Before we can see how such a theory might look, we need to get a little clearer about what consequentialism is in its barest form, once it has been divested of its familiar utilitarian garb. How, for instance, does it differ from non-consequentialist theories? The standard way of marking the distinction, of course, is something like this: "consequentialism is the view that acts are right or wrong in virtue of their consequences, or outcomes, while non-consequentialism is the view that acts are right or wrong in virtue of the kind of acts they are." By itself, this distinction is, as philosophers have been quick to point out, less than helpful.[2] One the one hand, surely the consequentialist too believes that an action is right or wrong in virtue of the kind of act it is: if it is the kind of act that has good consequences, then it is a right act. On the other hand, the non-consequentialist, in assessing an act, needs to take into account its consequences: as the problem of moral luck has forcefully shown us, what sort of act A is, is in part a function of A's outcome.[3] For example, A is not an act of killing unless one of A's consequences is that someone dies.

It would seem that a more satisfactory way of drawing the distinction is that adopted by, amongst others, Philip Pettit.[4] Pettit's claim is that whilst a consequentialist and a non-consequentialist theory may differ not at all in their accounts of the good, where they must differ—where the distinction between them lies—is in their accounts of the right. To explain: a theory T's account (or theory) of the right tells us what we ought to do in relation to the values that make up T's account (or theory) of the good. So, according to this way of drawing the distinction, we could have a consequentialist and a non-consequentialist theory that both held a commitment to realizing exactly the same values, or goods. Where they would diverge is in the way that they thought those values ought to be realized.

A consequentialist theory is one with an account of the right that tells us that we ought to *maximize* value. That is, in considering what we ought to do, we should opt for that course of action that will bring about most value in the world. So, in the case of a rights-based consequentialism, maximizing the value of rights will involve making sure that as many people's rights as possible are respected. At least, that is an exceedingly rough characterization of what it will involve. I will attempt to give a more precise characterization below.

A non-consequentialist theory's account of the right, by contrast, will tell us to *honor* values in our own actions. Where rights are among the values in question, this will mean making sure that we do not violate rights through our own actions. Crucially, such a theory will not allow what rights-based consequentialism will allow: it will not permit us to violate somebody's rights in order to ensure that more people's rights are respected. At least that is the claim, very roughly put. I will have reason to question it later.

What it means to say that our fledgling bioethicist has robust consequentialist intuitions, then, is that she feels that what is of value ought to be maximized. But she is not a utilitarian, because she believes that rights are among the things of non-derivative value that ought to be maximized.

It would be disingenuous to pretend that this way of marking the distinction between consequentialism and non-consequentialism is uncontroversial and uncontested. John Rawls, for instance, would have claimed that the introduction of rights into a moral theory's account of the good immediately renders that theory non-consequentialist. This is because rights, along with other "moral goods," such as the fair distribution of resources, fall under "the concept of right as one intuitively understands it, and so the theory lacks an independent definition of the good."[5] For Rawls, then, only non-moral goods—goods that can be characterized as such independently of any specification of what is right—can feature in an account of the good in a consequentialist theory.

I do not want to become embroiled in the issue of whether Rawls is right about this. I simply want to look at the prospects for a theory that tells us that rights are amongst the goods to be maximized, and I will refer to such a theory as a species of consequentialism, secure in the knowledge that at least some philosophers would categorize it as such.

Perhaps the most important question to be asked about such a theory at the outset is this: precisely what is it that the theory tells us to maximize? Earlier, in my rough characterization, I said that "maximizing the value of rights will involve making sure that as many people's rights as possible are respected." This is clearly nowhere near precise enough as it stands—all sorts of qualifications need to be added. Presumably, the diligent rights-based consequentialist would not think it right to ensure that three people could exercise a relatively trivial right, if to do so would involve the violation of one other person's right to life. So, we clearly need some sort of ranking of rights in order of importance, and some way of working out how many people need to benefit from having a right lower down in the hierarchy respected to justify one person's having a more important right violated. And the answer to this question will obviously not remain the same across all pairs of rights selected: for a particularly important right R, it may be the case that no amount of people benefiting from a lesser right's being respected could ever justify R's violation.

And the complexity does not end there. It might be claimed that some people have more right to have their rights respected than do others. For example, an average, law-abiding citizen might have more right to have her right to life respected than would a genocidal despot. If something about this claim sounds wrong, then perhaps it would be more accurate to say that in certain circumstances people, through their actions, can forfeit certain very important rights.

It is far beyond the scope of this chapter to set out a hierarchy of rights, to work out when lesser rights may override more important rights, or to say when a person forfeits certain rights, or does not deserve to have the rights she possesses taken into consideration. Instead, in what follows I will just suppose that we could formulate an acceptable account of what it would be to maximize respected rights, whilst acknowledging the obvious difficulties in doing so. In other words, I just want to assume that all the necessary qualifications, whatever they are, are taken as read in my claim that "maximizing the value of rights will involve making sure that as many people's rights as possible are respected." I will also sidestep any argument about whether what ought to be maximized is the number of respected rights, or the number of people with respected rights, and will assume that the second option is the more plausible.

Clearly, as a means to achieving this end, a rights-based consequentialism will also be concerned to maximize the number of people who respect rights. Bioethics is, of course, concerned with giving answers to moral problems encountered in medicine, bioscientific research, and related fields. So, it frequently suggests what policies ought to be adopted, for instance by hospital trusts, governments, and so on. This is not its exclusive use, and it may not even be its primary use, but it is perhaps the application with the most practical value, and it is certainly that which is most concerned with social reality. In such applications of bioethical method, the aim of the rights-based consequentialist will be to produce the policy that results in the maximum number of people with respected rights, from amongst that set of people who are users of the trust's services, who fall under the government's protection, and so on. That being the case, the person or body that formulates or implements a rights-based consequentialist policy will obliquely, or secondarily, be concerned to maximize, say, the number of agents of the trust who respect its users' rights.

In outline, then, a rights-based non-ultilitarian consequentialism will be one that affords rights an independent value—a value that is not dependent upon the contribution that respecting rights will make to the maximization of some other value (such as, in the case of utilitarianism, preference satisfaction). It will identify the right act or policy as being that, from the range of possible acts or policies, which will maximize, subject to numerous qualifications, the numbers of people with respected rights. I want now to turn to an important objection to theories of this sort.

3. An Unavoidable Tension Between Consequentialism and Rights?

There is much that is attractive about the theory sketched so far. If rights are possessed of an independent value, surely it can only be right to make sure that that value is maximized: that as many people as possible have their rights respected. However, it might be argued that to think in this way is to fail to grasp precisely what a right is, and why rights are so important. It may, that is, be urged that there is no compatibility between an account of the right that tells us to maximize value (the distinguishing feature, as we saw earlier, of a consequentialist theory), and an account of the good that posits rights as being of non-derivative, independent value. Behind this objection lies an intuition that it is quite hard to articulate with any great degree of precision, but which all the same has enormous force. It is the intuition that, in viewing someone as a bearer of rights, we are viewing her as essentially a separate, independent individual—a "world entire unto herself," in a much used phrase—who as such is not an appropriate item to be reduced to the status of a variable in calculations about what would maximize some good or other.

This intuition, of course, informs one of the standard objections levelled at utilitarianism by rights-theorists: the criticism that states that an individual's rights cannot legitimately be overridden in search of the general good. Indeed, it may seem that to have a right is, at least in part, to have a legitimate claim not to have certain of one's interests overridden in this way. An individual's rights cannot be sacrificed, for instance, just because to do so would lead to greater overall preference satisfaction, through the satisfaction of some comparatively trivial preferences being maximized.

This intuition, then, tells against utilitarianism: indeed, it is what drove our imaginary fledgling bioethicist, introduced in section one, to reject that theory. And it will also tell against a non-utilitarian consequentialism that gives rights an independent value, but that fails to place them at the top of its hierarchy of goods. To see what I mean by this, imagine a theory that gives both rights and happiness a non-derivative value, but in which rights have a value that is either lower than or equal to that afforded to happiness. In such a theory, five units of happiness will be seen as possessing greater value than four units of a right being respected, and considerations of happiness will consequently have the capacity to override consideration for individuals' rights. Indeed, they will also possess this capacity in a theory that places rights at the top of its hierarchy of goods, but in such a way that the aggregate happiness expected from a given action could be sufficiently large to justify rights being violated.

However, it is perfectly possible to construct a rights-based consequentialism in which rights are regarded as invariably able to trump all other goods. We can stipulate that it is a theory of this sort that our fledgling bioethicist finds most attractive. In such a theory, calculations about what ought to be done would only ever pit an individual's rights against the rights of others. Clearly, as mentioned above, among the rights that individuals may possess, there will be assumed to exist some sort of hierarchy—plainly some rights are more important than others. But when competing rights-claims *of the same level in the hierarchy* are viewed through a theory like this, we will simply have to make sure that as many people as possible have their rights respected. And, indeed, it is hard to see how the non-consequentialist rights-theorist could object to this. That is, there are circumstances in which *whatever we do*, somebody's rights will be violated. Let us call such circumstances "CR-circumstances," for "conflicting rights circumstances." If rights are valuable, as both the non-consequentialist and the rights-based consequentialist maintain, surely all that can be done in CR-circumstances is to maximize them. To put the point more forcefully: it seems that all we can do to honor rights in our own actions in CR-circumstances (the non-consequentialist requirement) is to maximize the number of people whose rights are respected (the rights-based consequentialist requirement). So it looks like the consequentialist and non-consequentialist theories collapse into each other whenever competing rights-claims appear on the horizon (at least where the competing rights are of the same level of importance).

It feels, though, as if the non-consequentialist should still be able to object to this. The rights-theorist's objection to consequentialism of any sort is that it clashes with the view of persons that underlies the attribution to them of rights. That view, as we have seen, is of persons as separate, unique individuals, "worlds entire unto themselves." The thought is that such persons ought not to be regarded as mere variables in calculations about what would maximize value, and we could argue that this remains the case *even when the value to be maximized is the number of people whose rights are respected.* Possessing rights legitimately exempts us from featuring in such calculations.

It seems correct to say that the reason there is a clash between the notion of maximization of value on the one hand, and the notion of a right on the other, is that while the first relies on what we can call an aggregative conception of value, the second depends on a radically non-aggregative view of persons. And it still might seem that we can appeal to this anti-aggregative view of a person, in order legitimately to exempt certain interests of hers—interests protected by rights—from being overridden by even directly comparable interests of a greater number of others. To amend a famous quotation of Rawls', all consequentialism, and not just the utilitarian variety, "does not take seriously the distinction between persons."[6] Perhaps the concept of a given right as something that a person holds equally with all others is able to help explicate this thought.

Suppose that the only way a particular agent A can safeguard a right R of ten people (call them B_1–B_{10}) is by failing to protect the right R of one person C. R is the same right in all eleven people. In deciding what she ought to do, A needs to consider that C's right R is held equally with each of B_1–B_{10}. The non-consequentialist of course agrees with this way of presenting the matter, but insists that A will go wrong if she assumes that the equality that holds between C and, say, B_1 means that C and B_1 each possess one unit of an aggregateable property that might be given the value 1, so that B_1–B_{10} collectively possess units with a value of 10. In other words, the non-consequentialist will say that the way in which an individual possesses R equally with all other bearers of R, means that the claim of C can only be considered against that of each of B_1–B_{10} individually, and not *en masse*.

The problem is that even if this point is coherent (which, incidentally, I think it is), it will not help much. That is, it still does not help us to decide whose right we ought to protect in a CR-circumstance like this, because such cases will always be equivalent to a conflict between two equal claims. As such, they will place us as agents in a position not dissimilar to that of Buridan's Ass (a donkey placed at an equal distance from two bales of hay, and consequently unable to decide which bale to eat). The non-consequentialist will need to take another tack if she is to keep her intuition intact.

The most promising tack, it seems to me, is this. We need to consider that, whatever else a right might be, it is a legitimate claim either to be treated in a certain way, or not to be treated in a certain way; to have certain things *done for us*, or not have certain things *done to us*. Note the essential reference here to the actions of others—no-one can have a right for something simply to happen to her, or not to happen to her; our rights are always claims on the *doings* of others. This is why they impose duties on others, obligations to do or not to do certain things.

Bearing that point in mind, imagine now that you are faced with one person, and that failure to violate some right R of that one person would involve failure to protect the same right R of ten others. What ought you to do? Well, whatever you do, you will be doing to that one person in front of you. If you violate a right of hers, it is pretty clear that you will have used her as a means of protecting the rights of ten others. But the way of looking at persons that conceives of each as a world entire unto herself, each with her own distinct value, will condemn this way of acting. She herself will have reason to complain about the way you have treated her: you have failed to treat her as the separate, individually valuable being she is. You have, in the Kantian sense, treated her as a means only, and not as an end in herself.

But what of the other ten people caught up in this CR-circumstance? Will it not be the case that you have also treated them inappropriately if you protect the one person's rights? Well, on one understanding, you will not have treated them badly, since you will not have *treated* them in any way at all. Nothing has been done to them, at least not by you; instead, at least from your perspective, something has happened to them. That being the case, it is, strictly speaking, inaccurate to say that any rights of theirs have been violated; instead, it is just the case that something bad has happened to them. This is a version of a point made by Thomas Nagel and, as Nagel acknowledges, it involves commitment to a principle which is at least clearly related to, if not identical with, the doctrine of double-effect.[7]

This, then, appears to be the most plausible way of unpacking the anti-aggregationism intuition. But is it really convincing? Can we really be said, in our imagined situation, not to have done something to the unfortunate ten, and so not to have violated their rights? I must confess that my own answer to this question has, at least at the time of writing, a distressing tendency to vary. However, the important point is that I am not, for the purposes of this chapter, obliged to arrive at a definite answer, because when we try to apply what has been said to a vitally important subset of bioethical problems—those that demand an answer that can inform policy—it becomes significantly irrelevant.

4. Rights-Maximizing Policies, and the Collapse of a Distinction

What is the social benefit of work in bioethics? What has bioethics to do with social reality? The answer to these questions, already given earlier in this chapter, would appear to be that it can guide the formulation of policies. It is to be hoped, that is, that it can produce answers to the question of what policies governments, health services, and so on, ought to adopt. Now, policy-makers, *qua* policy-makers, do not find themselves in the sort of position described in my "one-to-ten" example. They are not immediately presented with one person with a particular right, a person who stands in the moral foreground, while others with conflicting rights lurk somewhere out of sight in the moral background. Indeed, they are not usually immediately presented with anyone. But what they do in making policy, they do to potentially huge numbers of people, among whom there may exist conflicting rights. For example, they may have to construct policies about the distribution of scarce resources, resources to which all affected by the policy have an equal right. It seems to me that in CR-circumstances such as this, the policy maker has no choice but to maximize the number of people whose rights are respected. What else can she do? There simply is no practical alternative at the vantage point from which she is forced to make her decision—a vantage point where all those affected by her decision stand equally in the moral foreground, where all are having something done to them. Some recommended course of action is necessary, and there seems to be no other basis for it than aggregative calculation.

It is highly significant that, when all are in the moral foreground in this way, it does not much matter whether the policy maker's action is described as maximizing the number of people whose rights are respected, or whether the policy maker is described as honoring rights in her own action. That is, it seems that the only way in which she is able to honor rights in her own action is by maximizing the number of people whose rights are respected. So, again the non-consequentialist and rights-based consequentialist approaches collapse into each other, and this time no moral foreground-background distinction is available to prevent that collapse. It is not simply that they produce the same answers, but that they become genuinely indistinguishable from each other.

5. The Puzzle

There is something really quite unsatisfactory about the collapse of the distinction between consequentialist and non-consequentialist approaches to rights when making policies that cover CR-circumstances. It is not simply that we do not, when making or recommending such policies, appear to be able to stick rigorously to our preferred moral theory. Indeed, we can if we want still maintain that we are either consequentialists or non-consequentialists even here—the consequentialist can say that she is honoring rights in her action *because* that involves maximizing their respect. And the non-consequentialist can say that she is maximizing respected rights only *because* that is the way, in this situation, to honor them in her own action. Instead, the dissatisfaction arises because the claim that the notion of a right rests upon a radically non-aggregative conception of persons appears to be correct.

To claim a right is to claim, so far as the interest protected by that right is concerned, legitimate exemption from being counted as the value of a variable in aggregative calculations that aim at the maximization of goods. Now, since in CR-circumstances the perspective of the bioethical policy-maker can only lead to rights being honored through the number of people whose rights are respected being maximized, it seems that that perspective is curiously blind to what is essentially involved in the notion of a right. We might say that theories that aim only to maximize values can never *really* include rights in their list of the values to be maximized: only the simulacra of rights can be included in their accounts of the good.[8] But then since the only way of honoring rights in the formation of policies is to seek to maximize them, and since to seek to maximize rights is to lose sight of what a right essentially is, it would appear to be impossible really to honor rights in the formulation of policies.

I suppose we might just want to bite the bullet and say that this is the case. We could say that the policy-maker is not aiming at maximizing respected rights at all in CR-circumstances, but is instead aiming at maximizing the goods to which those rights entitle people. And while this redescription might make her actions sound a little less noble, it has to be admitted that those goods are tremendously important. Indeed, they are so important that people have rights to them.

Would this be a satisfactory route to take? I do not think that it would. If a right is a legitimate claim not to be featured in calculations about what would maximize some good or other (including the good of rights being respected), then it would appear that its true usefulness shows itself just when people are making such calculations. Ideally, the thought that someone has a right in such situations ought to act as a "brake," the application of which ensures that she is not treated as a mere variable in the right-maximizing equation. And such a brake is needed in CR-circumstances just as much as it is in circumstances in which rights come into conflict with lesser goods. That being the case, it is especially frustrating and puzzling that the non-aggregative view of persons that underlies the notion of a right should of necessity become unavailable just at the moment when it becomes most needed. This, then, is the paradox to which our thoughts about rights-based consequentialism have led: that the distinction between rights-based consequentialism and non-consequentialism collapses just when its being drawn becomes most important.

NOTES

1. Anne Maclean, *The Elimination of Morality: Reflections on Utilitarianism and Bioethics* (London: Routledge, 1993).

2. E.g. Roger Crisp, "Ethics in the Modern World," *New British Philosophy: The Interviews*, Julian Baggini and Jeremy Stangroom, eds. (London: Routledge, 2002), pp. 31–32.

3. Thomas Nagel, "Moral Luck," *Mortal Questions* (New York, NY: Cambridge University Press, 1979)

4. Philip Pettit, "Consequentialism," *A Companion to Ethics*, Peter Singer, ed. (Oxford: Blackwell Publishers, 1991), pp. 230–240.

5. John Rawls, *A Theory of Justice* (Oxford: Oxford University Press, 1999), p. 22.

6. *Ibid.*, p. 24.

7. Thomas Nagel, "Autonomy and Deontology," *Consequentialism and its Critics*, Samuel Scheffler, ed. (Oxford: Oxford University Press, 1988), pp. 142-172.

8. See Samuel Scheffler, "Introduction," *Consequentialism and its Critics*, Samuel Scheffler, ed. (New York, NY: Oxford University Press, 1988), p. 2.

ABOUT THE EDITORS AND CONTRIBUTORS

Angus Dawson is currently Director of the Centre for Professional Ethics at Keele University. His main research interests are in public health ethics and the interaction between empirical and normative issues. His paper in this collection is one in a series he is writing looking at the implications of empirical evidence for different ethical arguments about informed consent. He has also written about these issues in relation to research ethics.

Eve Garrard is Senior Lecturer in Ethics and Philosophy in the Centre for Professional Ethics at Keele University. Before moving to Keele, she worked for several years for the Open University, and has a strong interest in teaching philosophy to adult beginning students. Much of her teaching is now to healthcare (and other) professionals. Her research interests are in moral theory and applied ethics, including bioethics, and also philosophical issues arising out of the Holocaust. She has recently published papers on the nature of evil and forgiveness.

Matti Häyry is Head of the Centre for Professional Ethics and Professor of Moral Philosophy at the University of Central Lancashire. He has taught philosophy and bioethics in various Finnish Universities since 1985, and co-ordinated research projects in bioethics at the University of Helsinki. He has been a permanent adviser on bioethics to the Finnish National Research and Development Center for Welfare and Health since 1991, and has participated in the work of legislative committees at the Finnish Ministries of Justice and Health. His publications include *Critical Studies in Philosophical Medical Ethics* (1990), *Liberal Utilitarianism and Applied Ethics* (1994, 2002), *Playing God: Essays on Bioethics* (2001), and many articles on bioethics and general philosophy in academic journals and edited collections.

Peter Herissone-Kelly is Lecturer in Professional Ethics in the Centre for Professional Ethics at the University of Central Lancashire, UK. He has a B.A. in Philosophy from Bolton Institute, a B.Phil. in Philosophy from the University of Oxford, and a background in philosophical logic and metaphysics. He is currently working on a Ph.D. thesis to be entitled *Kant on Rational Agency.*

Søren Holm is Professorial Fellow in Bioethics at Cardiff University, and Professor of Medical Ethics at the University of Oslo. He holds degrees in medicine, philosophy and healthcare ethics, and two doctoral degrees. He is a former member of the Danish Council of Ethics, which advises the Danish Government and Parliament on bioethical issues.

Louise Irving is Research Associate on the European Commission funded EUROSTEM Project, which seeks to develop an ethical framework for human stem cell research. She has written on the commodification of the human body, the nature of genetic information, the relationship between analytic moral philosophy and bioethics, and ethical dilemmas in IVF and bio-banking. Her main interest is in the relationship between freedom and language.

Monique Jonas is a Lecturer in Ethics at Keele University, UK. Her research interests include ethical problems in decision making for children, property theory and bioethics, and the relationship between ethics and public policy. She has co-edited a volume of essays on the role of empirical research in bioethics and the regulation of biotechnologies with Søren Holm.

Jukka Kilpi is Docent of Business Ethics at the University of Turku, Finland and Visiting Fellow at the Centre for Professional Ethics, University of Central Lancashire, UK. He is also CEO of the Finland-based corporate finance consulting company Kapai Oy, and an Associate of the Securities Institute of Australia. Dr Kilpi's book *The Ethics of Bankruptcy* is published in Routledge's Professional Ethics series. He has numerous articles in books and journals including the *Encyclopedia of Applied Ethics*, *Australasian Journal of Philosophy*, *Public Affairs Quarterly* and *Journal of Business Ethics*.

Harry Lesser is a Senior Lecturer in Philosophy at the University of Manchester. He is author of several articles in the field of Medical Ethics, some being in journals and some being contributions to books, and editor of the collection *Ageing, Autonomy, and Resources* (Ashgate, 1999). He has particular interests, in both teaching and research, in the philosophy of psychiatry, and in issues concerning ageing and the elderly. He is currently working on papers on personal identity and dementia, and on research on the quality of life in old age. He is also editing a collection of papers entitled *Justice and Ageing*, to be published by Rodopi.

Peter Lucas is Lecturer in Bioethics at the Centre for Professional Ethics, the University of Central Lancashire, UK. His research interests include virtue ethics, risk and the public understanding of science, post-phenomenological continental philosophy, and critical theory. He has previously contributed articles to *Environmental Ethics*, *Environmental Values and Philosophy of the Social Sciences*.

Doris Schroeder was educated in Germany and the United Kingdom at postgraduate level in economics/management and philosophy/politics. She worked as a Lecturer in Philosophy at Lancaster University and currently holds the post of Senior Lecturer in Philosophy at the Centre for Professional Ethics in Preston, UK. Her book publications include, *Work Incentives and Welfare Provision—The Pathological Theory of Unemployment* (2000), *Applied Ethics*, a collection in six volumes co-edited with Ruth Chadwick (2002), and *Functional Foods*, co-authored with Ruth Chadwick *et al* (2003).

Mark Sheehan is a Lecturer in Philosophy and applied ethics in the Centre for Professional Ethics at Keele University. His main research interests are in metaethics, "metabioethics," research ethics, and resource allocation issues. His most recent publications include a pair of articles on practical reasoning in primary care for the *British Journal of General Practice*, and a paper on "the social reality of health" in a volume on distributive justice and healthcare.

Tuija Takala is Docent in Practical Philosophy at the University of Helsinki, Finland and Lecturer in Bioethics at the University of Manchester. She has taught philosophy at the Universities of Helsinki and Kuopio in Finland. Her research interests include political philosophy and applied ethics, particularly bioethics. Her publications include *Genes, Sense, and Sensibility: Philosophical Studies on the Ethics of Modern Biotechnologies* (2000), Scratching the Surface of Bioethics (edited with Matti Häyry, 2003) and articles in *Bioethics*, *Cambridge Quarterly of Healthcare Ethics*, *Journal of Medical Ethics*, *The Journal of Medicine and Philosophy*, and *Theoretical Medicine and Bioethics*.

Stephen Wilkinson is Senior Lecturer in Ethics and Philosophy in the Centre for Professional Ethics at Keele University. His research papers have addressed topics including the allocation of health service resources, selective savior siblings, separating conjoined twins, and the nature of mental illness. A paper on this last topic won the *Philosophical Quarterly* International Essay Prize in 1999. He has recently completed a book on the ethics of commercializing the human body (*Bodies for Sale*, Routledge, 2003) and is Program Director of Keele's new professional doctorate in Medical Ethics, the D.Med.Eth, as well as of its long-standing M.A. in Medical Ethics and Law.

Simon Woods is a Senior Lecturer at the Policy, Ethics, and Life Sciences Research Institute (PEALS), University of Newcastle, UK, where he is the Director of Learning and works closely with the Life Knowledge Park—one of the six national Genetics Knowledge Parks recently established in the UK. He is also a Fellow of the Institute of Medicine Law and Bioethics at the University of Manchester, is qualified as a nurse, and holds bachelor's and doctoral degrees in Philosophy. He has conducted both empirical and conceptual research, and has published widely in healthcare ethics.

INDEX

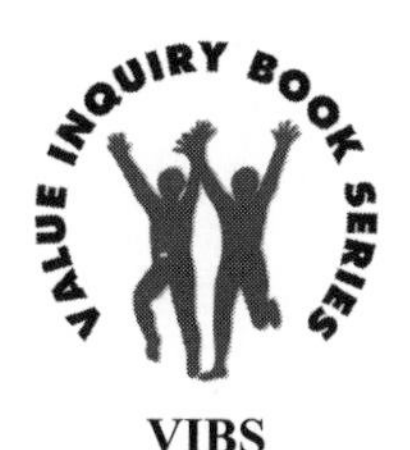

VIBS

The **Value Inquiry Book Series** is co-sponsored by:

Adler School of Professional Psychology
American Indian Philosophy Association
American Maritain Association
American Society for Value Inquiry
Association for Process Philosophy of Education
Canadian Society for Philosophical Practice
Center for Bioethics, University of Turku
Center for Professional and Applied Ethics, University of North Carolina at Charlotte
Central European Pragmatist Forum
Centre for Applied Ethics, Hong Kong Baptist University
Centre for Cultural Research, Aarhus University
Centre for Professional Ethics, University of Central Lancashire
Centre for the Study of Philosophy and Religion, University College of Cape Breton
Centro de Estudos em Filosofia Americana, Brazil
College of Education and Allied Professions, Bowling Green State University
College of Liberal Arts, Rochester Institute of Technology
Concerned Philosophers for Peace
Conference of Philosophical Societies
Department of Moral and Social Philosophy, University of Helsinki
Gannon University
Gilson Society
Haitian Studies Association
Ikeda University
Institute of Philosophy of the High Council of Scientific Research, Spain
International Academy of Philosophy of the Principality of Liechtenstein
International Association of Bioethics
International Center for the Arts, Humanities, and Value Inquiry
International Society for Universal Dialogue
Natural Law Society
Philosophical Society of Finland
Philosophy Born of Struggle Association
Philosophy Seminar, University of Mainz
Pragmatism Archive at The Oklahoma State University
R.S. Hartman Institute for Formal and Applied Axiology
Research Institute, Lakeridge Health Corporation
Russian Philosophical Society
Society for Iberian and Latin-American Thought
Society for the Philosophic Study of Genocide and the Holocaust
Unit for Research in Cognitive Neuroscience, Autonomous University of Barcelona
Yves R. Simon Institute

Titles Published

1. Noel Balzer, *The Human Being as a Logical Thinker*

2. Archie J. Bahm, *Axiology: The Science of Values*

3. H. P. P. (Hennie) Lötter, *Justice for an Unjust Society*

4. H. G. Callaway, *Context for Meaning and Analysis: A Critical Study in the Philosophy of Language*

5. Benjamin S. Llamzon, *A Humane Case for Moral Intuition*

6. James R. Watson, *Between Auschwitz and Tradition: Postmodern Reflections on the Task of Thinking.* A volume in **Holocaust and Genocide Studies**

7. Robert S. Hartman, *Freedom to Live: The Robert Hartman Story*, Edited by Arthur R. Ellis. A volume in **Hartman Institute Axiology Studies**

8. Archie J. Bahm, *Ethics: The Science of Oughtness*

9. George David Miller, *An Idiosyncratic Ethics; Or, the Lauramachean Ethics*

10. Joseph P. DeMarco, *A Coherence Theory in Ethics*

11. Frank G. Forrest, *Valuemetrics*[ℵ]: *The Science of Personal and Professional Ethics.* A volume in **Hartman Institute Axiology Studies**

12. William Gerber, *The Meaning of Life: Insights of the World's Great Thinkers*

13. Richard T. Hull, Editor, *A Quarter Century of Value Inquiry: Presidential Addresses of the American Society for Value Inquiry*. A volume in **Histories and Addresses of Philosophical Societies**

14. William Gerber, *Nuggets of Wisdom from Great Jewish Thinkers: From Biblical Times to the Present*

15. Sidney Axinn, *The Logic of Hope: Extensions of Kant's View of Religion*

16. Messay Kebede, *Meaning and Development*

17. Amihud Gilead, *The Platonic Odyssey: A Philosophical-Literary Inquiry into the Phaedo*

18. Necip Fikri Alican, *Mill's Principle of Utility: A Defense of John Stuart Mill's Notorious Proof.* A volume in **Universal Justice**

19. Michael H. Mitias, Editor, *Philosophy and Architecture.*

20. Roger T. Simonds, *Rational Individualism: The Perennial Philosophy of Legal Interpretation.* A volume in **Natural Law Studies**

21. William Pencak, The Conflict of Law and Justice in the Icelandic Sagas

22. Samuel M. Natale and Brian M. Rothschild, Editors, *Values, Work, Education: The Meanings of Work*

23. N. Georgopoulos and Michael Heim, Editors, *Being Human in the Ultimate: Studies in the Thought of John M. Anderson*

24. Robert Wesson and Patricia A. Williams, Editors, *Evolution and Human* Values

25. Wim J. van der Steen, *Facts, Values, and Methodology: A New Approach to Ethics*

26. Avi Sagi and Daniel Statman, *Religion and Morality*

27. Albert William Levi, *The High Road of Humanity: The Seven Ethical Ages of Western Man*, Edited by Donald Phillip Verene and Molly Black Verene

28. Samuel M. Natale and Brian M. Rothschild, Editors, *Work Values: Education, Organization, and Religious Concerns*

29. Laurence F. Bove and Laura Duhan Kaplan, Editors, *From the Eye of the Storm: Regional Conflicts and the Philosophy of Peace.* A volume in **Philosophy of Peace**

30. Robin Attfield, *Value, Obligation, and Meta-Ethics*

31. William Gerber, *The Deepest Questions You Can Ask About God: As Answered by the World's Great Thinkers*

32. Daniel Statman, *Moral Dilemmas*

33. Rem B. Edwards, Editor, *Formal Axiology and Its Critics*. A volume in **Hartman Institute Axiology Studies**

34. George David Miller and Conrad P. Pritscher, *On Education and Values: In Praise of Pariahs and Nomads*. A volume in **Philosophy of Education**

35. Paul S. Penner, *Altruistic Behavior: An Inquiry into Motivation*

36. Corbin Fowler, *Morality for Moderns*

37. Giambattista Vico, *The Art of Rhetoric* (*Institutiones Oratoriae*, 1711–1741), from the definitive Latin text and notes, Italian commentary and introduction byGiuliano Crifò.Translated and Edited by Giorgio A. Pinton and Arthur W. Shippee. A volume in **Values in Italian Philosophy**

38. W. H. Werkmeister, *Martin Heidegger on the Way*. Edited by Richard T. Hull. A volume in **Werkmeister Studies**

39. Phillip Stambovsky, *Myth and the Limits of Reason*

40. Samantha Brennan, Tracy Isaacs, and Michael Milde, Editors, *A Question of Values: New Canadian Perspectives in Ethics and Political Philosophy*

41. Peter A. Redpath, *Cartesian Nightmare: An Introduction to Transcendental Sophistry*. A volume in **Studies in the History of Western Philosophy**

42. Clark Butler, *History as the Story of Freedom: Philosophy in InterculturalContext*, with responses by sixteen scholars

43. Dennis Rohatyn, *Philosophy History Sophistry*

44. Leon Shaskolsky Sheleff, *Social Cohesion and Legal Coercion: A Critique of Weber, Durkheim, and Marx*. Afterword by Virginia Black

45. Alan Soble, Editor, *Sex, Love, and Friendship: Studies of the Society for the Philosophy of Sex and Love, 1977–1992*. A volume in **Histories and Addresses of Philosophical Societies**

46. Peter A. Redpath, *Wisdom's Odyssey: From Philosophy to Transcendental Sophistry*. A volume in **Studies in the History of Western Philosophy**

47. Albert A. Anderson, *Universal Justice: A Dialectical Approach*. A volume in **Universal Justice**

48. Pio Colonnello, *The Philosophy of José Gaos*. Translated from Italian by Peter Cocozzella. Edited by Myra Moss. Introduction by Giovanni Gullace. A volume in **Values in Italian Philosophy**

49. Laura Duhan Kaplan and Laurence F. Bove, Editors, *Philosophical Perspectives on Power and Domination: Theories and Practices*. A volume in **Philosophy of Peace**

50. Gregory F. Mellema, *Collective Responsibility*

51. Josef Seifert, *What Is Life? The Originality, Irreducibility, and Value of Life*. A volume in **Central-European Value Studies**

52. William Gerber, *Anatomy of What We Value Most*

53. Armando Molina, *Our Ways: Values and Character*, Edited by Rem B. Edwards. A volume in **Hartman Institute Axiology Studies**

54. Kathleen J. Wininger, *Nietzsche's Reclamation of Philosophy*. A volume in **Central-European Value Studies**

55. Thomas Magnell, Editor, *Explorations of Value*

56. HPP (Hennie) Lötter, *Injustice, Violence, and Peace: The Case of South Africa*. A volume in **Philosophy of Peace**

57. Lennart Nordenfelt, *Talking About Health: A Philosophical Dialogue*. A volume in **Nordic Value Studies**

58. Jon Mills and Janusz A. Polanowski, *The Ontology of Prejudice*. A volume in **Philosophy and Psychology**

59. Leena Vilkka, *The Intrinsic Value of Nature*

60. Palmer Talbutt, Jr., Rough Dialectics: *Sorokin's Philosophy of Value*, with contributions by Lawrence T. Nichols and Pitirim A. Sorokin

61. C. L. Sheng, *A Utilitarian General Theory of Value*

62. George David Miller, *Negotiating Toward Truth: The Extinction of Teachers and Students*. Epilogue by Mark Roelof Eleveld. A volume in **Philosophy of Education**

63. William Gerber, *Love, Poetry, and Immortality: Luminous Insights of the World's Great Thinkers*

64. Dane R. Gordon, Editor, *Philosophy in Post-Communist Europe*. A volume in **Post-Communist European Thought**

65. Dane R. Gordon and Józef Niznik, Editors, *Criticism and Defense of Rationality in Contemporary Philosophy*. A volume in **Post-Communist European Thought**

66. John R. Shook, *Pragmatism: An Annotated Bibliography, 1898-1940*. With contributions by E. Paul Colella, Lesley Friedman, Frank X. Ryan, and Ignas K. Skrupskelis

67. Lansana Keita, *The Human Project and the Temptations of Science*

68. Michael M. Kazanjian, *Phenomenology and Education: Cosmology, Co-Being, and Core Curriculum*. A volume in **Philosophy of Education**

69. James W. Vice, *The Reopening of the American Mind: On Skepticism and Constitutionalism*

70. Sarah Bishop Merrill, *Defining Personhood: Toward the Ethics of Quality in Clinical Care*

71. Dane R. Gordon, *Philosophy and Vision*

72. Alan Milchman and Alan Rosenberg, Editors, *Postmodernism and the Holocaust*. A volume in **Holocaust and Genocide Studies**

73. Peter A. Redpath, *Masquerade of the Dream Walkers: Prophetic Theology from the Cartesians to Hegel*. A volume in **Studies in the History of Western Philosophy**

74. Malcolm D. Evans, *Whitehead and Philosophy of Education: The Seamless Coat of Learning*. A volume in **Philosophy of Education**

75. Warren E. Steinkraus, *Taking Religious Claims Seriously: A Philosophy of Religion*, Edited by Michael H. Mitias. A volume in **Universal Justice**

76. Thomas Magnell, Editor, *Values and Education*

77. Kenneth A. Bryson, *Persons and Immortality*. A volume in **Natural Law Studies**

78. Steven V. Hicks, *International Law and the Possibility of a Just World Order: An Essay on Hegel's Universalism*. A volume in **Universal Justice**

79. E. F. Kaelin, *Texts on Texts and Textuality: A Phenomenology of Literary Art*, Edited by Ellen J. Burns

80. Amihud Gilead, *Saving Possibilities: A Study in Philosophical Psychology*. A volume in Philosophy and Psychology

81. André Mineau, *The Making of the Holocaust: Ideology and Ethics in the Systems Perspective*. A volume in **Holocaust and Genocide Studies**

82. Howard P. Kainz, *Politically Incorrect Dialogues: Topics Not Discussed in Polite Circles*

83. Veikko Launis, Juhani Pietarinen, and Juha Räikkä, Editors, *Genes and Morality: New Essays*. A volume in **Nordic Value Studies**

84. Steven Schroeder, *The Metaphysics of Cooperation: A Study of F. D. Maurice*

85. Caroline Joan ("Kay") S. Picart, *Thomas Mann and Friedrich Nietzsche: Eroticism, Death, Music, and Laughter*. A volume in **Central-European Value Studies**

86. G. John M. Abbarno, Editor, *The Ethics of Homelessness: Philosophical Perspectives*

87. James Giles, Editor, *French Existentialism: Consciousness, Ethics, and Relations with Others*. A volume in **Nordic Value Studies**

88. Deane Curtin and Robert Litke, Editors, *Institutional Violence*. A volume in **Philosophy of Peace**

89. Yuval Lurie, *Cultural Beings: Reading the Philosophers of Genesis*

90. Sandra A. Wawrytko, Editor, *The Problem of Evil: An Intercultural Exploration.* A volume in **Philosophy and Psychology**

91. Gary J. Acquaviva, *Values, Violence, and Our Future*. A volume in **Hartman Institute Axiology Studies**

92. Michael R. Rhodes, *Coercion: A Nonevaluative Approach*

93. Jacques Kriel, *Matter, Mind, and Medicine: Transforming the Clinical Method*

94. Haim Gordon, *Dwelling Poetically: Educational Challenges in Heidegger's Thinking on Poetry*. A volume in **Philosophy of Education**

95. Ludwig Grünberg, *The Mystery of Values: Studies in Axiology*, Edited by Cornelia Grünberg and Laura Grünberg

96. Gerhold K. Becker, Editor, *The Moral Status of Persons: Perspectives on Bioethics*. A volume in **Studies in Applied Ethics**

97. Roxanne Claire Farrar, *Sartrean Dialectics: A Method for Critical Discourse on Aesthetic Experience*

98. Ugo Spirito, *Memoirs of the Twentieth Century*. Translated from Italian and Edited by Anthony G. Costantini. A volume in **Values in Italian Philosophy**

99. Steven Schroeder, *Between Freedom and Necessity: An Essay on the Place of Value*

100. Foster N. Walker, *Enjoyment and the Activity of Mind: Dialogues on Whitehead and Education*. A volume in **Philosophy of Education**

101. Avi Sagi, Kierkegaard, *Religion, and Existence: The Voyage of the Self*. Translated from Hebrew by Batya Stein

102. Bennie R. Crockett, Jr., Editor, *Addresses of the Mississippi Philosophical Association*. A volume in **Histories and Addresses of Philosophical Societies**

103. Paul van Dijk, *Anthropology in the Age of Technology: The Philosophical Contribution of Günther Anders*

104. Giambattista Vico, *Universal Right*. Translated from Latin and edited by Giorgio Pinton and Margaret Diehl. A volume in **Values in Italian Philosophy**

105. Judith Presler and Sally J. Scholz, Editors, *Peacemaking: Lessons from the Past, Visions for the Future*. A volume in **Philosophy of Peace**

106. Dennis Bonnette, *Origin of the Human Species*. A volume in **Studies in the History of Western Philosophy**

107. Phyllis Chiasson, *Peirce's Pragmatism: The Design for Thinking*. A volume in **Studies in Pragmatism and Values**

108. Dan Stone, Editor, *Theoretical Interpretations of the Hol*ocaust. A volume in **Holocaust and Genocide Studies**

109. Raymond Angelo Belliotti, *What Is the Meaning of Human Life?*

110. Lennart Nordenfelt, *Health, Science, and Ordinary Language*, with Contributions by George Khushf and K. W. M. Fulford

111. Daryl Koehn, *Local Insights, Global Ethics for Business*. A volume in **Studies in Applied Ethics**

112. Matti Häyry and Tuija Takala, Editors, *The Future of Value Inquiry*. A volume in **Nordic Value Studies**

113. Conrad P. Pritscher, *Quantum Learning: Beyond Duality*

114. Thomas M. Dicken and Rem B. Edwards, *Dialogues on Values and Centers of Value: Old Friends, New Thoughts*. A volume in **Hartman Institute Axiology Studies**

115. Rem B. Edwards, *What Caused the Big Bang?* A volume in **Philosophy and Religion**

116. Jon Mills, Editor, *A Pedagogy of Becoming*. A volume in **Philosophy of Education**

117. Robert T. Radford, *Cicero: A Study in the Origins of Republican Philosophy*. A volume in **Studies in the History of Western Philosophy**

118. Arleen L. F. Salles and María Julia Bertomeu, Editors, *Bioethics: Latin American Perspectives*. A volume in **Philosophy in Latin America**

119. Nicola Abbagnano, *The Human Project: The Year 2000*, with an Interview by Guiseppe Grieco. Translated from Italian by Bruno Martini and Nino Langiulli. Edited with an introduction by Nino Langiulli. A volume in **Studies in the History of Western Philosophy**

120. Daniel M. Haybron, Editor, *Earth's Abominations: Philosophical Studies of Evil*. A volume in **Personalist Studies**

121. Anna T. Challenger, *Philosophy and Art in Gurdjieff's* Beelzebub*: A Modern Sufi Odyssey*

122. George David Miller, *Peace, Value, and Wisdom: The Educational Philosophy of Daisaku Ikeda*. A volume in **Daisaku Ikeda Studies**

123. Haim Gordon and Rivca Gordon, *Sophistry and Twentieth-Century Art*

124. Thomas O. Buford and Harold H. Oliver, Editors *Personalism Revisited: Its Proponents and Critics*. A volume in **Histories and Addresses of Philosophical Societies**

125. Avi Sagi, *Albert Camus and the Philosophy of the Absurd*. Translated from Hebrew by Batya Stein

126. Robert S. Hartman, *The Knowledge of Good: Critique of Axiological Reason*. Expanded translation from the Spanish by Robert S. Hartman. Edited by Arthur R. Ellis and Rem B. Edwards.A volume in **Hartman Institute Axiology Studies**

127. Alison Bailey and Paula J. Smithka, Editors. *Community, Diversity, and Difference: Implications for Peace.* A volume in **Philosophy of Peace**

128. Oscar Vilarroya, *The Dissolution of Mind: A Fable of How Experience Gives Rise to Cognition.* A volume in **Cognitive Science**

129. Paul Custodio Bube and Jeffery Geller, Editors, *Conversations with Pragmatism: A Multi-Disciplinary Study.* A volume in **Studies in Pragmatism and Values**

130. Richard Rumana, *Richard Rorty: An Annotated Bibliography of Secondary Literature.* A volume in **Studies in Pragmatism and Values**

131. Stephen Schneck, Editor, *Max Scheler's Acting Persons: New Perspectives* A volume in **Personalist Studies**

132. Michael Kazanjian, *Learning Values Lifelong: From Inert Ideas to Wholes.* A volume in **Philosophy of Education**

133. Rudolph Alexander Kofi Cain, Alain Leroy Locke: *Race, Culture, and the Education of African American Adults.* A volume in **African American Philosophy**

134. Werner Krieglstein, *Compassion: A New Philosophy of the Other*

135. Robert N. Fisher, Daniel T. Primozic, Peter A. Day, and Joel A. Thompson, Editors, *Suffering, Death, and Identity.* A volume in **Personalist Studies**

136. Steven Schroeder, *Touching Philosophy, Sounding Religion, Placing Education.* A volume in **Philosophy of Education**

137. Guy DeBrock, *Process Pragmatism: Essays on a Quiet Philosophical Revolution.* A volume in **Studies in Pragmatism and Values**

138. Lennart Nordenfelt and Per-Erik Liss, Editors, *Dimensions of Health and Health Promotion*

139. Amihud Gilead, *Singularity and Other Possibilities: Panenmentalist Novelties*

140. Samantha Mei-che Pang, *Nursing Ethics in Modern China: Conflicting Values and Competing Role Requirements*. A volume in **Studies in Applied Ethics**

141. Christine M. Koggel, Allannah Furlong, and Charles Levin, Editors, *Confidential Relationships: Psychoanalytic, Ethical, and Legal Contexts*. A volume in **Philosophy and Psychology**

142. Peter A. Redpath, Editor, *A Thomistic Tapestry: Essays in Memory of Étienne Gilson*. A volume in **Gilson Studies**

143. Deane-Peter Baker and Patrick Maxwell, Editors, *Explorations in Contemporary Continental Philosophy of Religion*. A volume in **Philosophy and Religion**

144. Matti Häyry and Tuija Takala, Editors, *Scratching the Surface of Bioethics*. A volume in **Values in Bioethics**

145. Leonidas Donskis, *Forms of Hatred: The Troubled Imagination in Modern Philosophy and Literature*

146. Andreea Deciu Ritivoi, Editor, *Interpretation and Its Objects: Studies in the Philosophy of Michael Krausz*

147. Herman Stark, *A Fierce Little Tragedy: Thought, Passion, and Self-Formation in the Philosophy Classroom*. A volume in **Philosophy of Education**

148. William Gay and Tatiana Alekseeva, Editors, *Democracy and the Quest for Justice: Russian and American Perspectives*. A volume in **Contemporary Russian Philosophy**

149. Xunwu Chen, *Being and Authenticity*

150. Hugh P. McDonald, *Radical Axiology: A First Philosophy of Values*

151. Dane R. Gordon and David C. Durst, Editors, *Civil Society in Southeast Europe*. A volume in **Post-Communist European Thought**

152. John Ryder and Emil Višňovský, Editors, *Pragmatism and Values: The Central European Pragmatist Forum, Volume One*. A volume in **Studies in Pragmatism and Values**

153. Messay Kebede, *Africa's Quest for a Philosophy of Decolonization*

154. Steven M. Rosen, *Dimensions of* Apeiron: *A Topological Phenomenology of Space, Time, and Individuation*. A volume in **Philosophy and Psychology**

155. Albert A. Anderson, Steven V. Hicks, and Lech Witkowski, Editors, *Mythos and Logos: How to Regain the Love of Wisdom*. A volume in **Universal Justice**

156. John Ryder and Krystyna Wilkoszewska, Editors, *Deconstruction and Reconstruction: The Central European Pragmatist Forum, Volume Two*. A volume in **Studies in Pragmatism and Values**

157. Javier Muguerza, *Ethics and Perplexity: Toward a Critique of Dialogical Reason*. Translated from the Spanish by Jody L. Doran. Edited by John R. Welch. A volume in **Philosophy in Spain**

158. Gregory F. Mellema, *The Expectations of Morality*

159. Robert Ginsberg, *The Aesthetics of Ruins*

160. Stan van Hooft, *Life, Death, and Subjectivity: Moral Sources in Bioethics* A volume in **Values in Bioethics**

161. André Mineau, *Operation Barbarossa: Ideology and Ethics Against Human Dignity*

162. Arthur Efron, *Expriencing Tess of the D'Urbervilles: A Deweyan Account.* A volume in **Studies in Pragmatism and Values**

163. Reyes Mate, *Memory of the West: The Contemporaneity of Forgotten Jewish Thinkers.* Translated from the Spanish by Anne Day Dewey. Edited by John R. Welch. A volume in **Philosophy in Spain**

164. Nancy Nyquist Potter, Editor, *Putting Peace into Practice: Evaluating Policy on Local and Global Levels.* A volume in **Philosophy of Peace**

165. Matti Häyry, Tuija Takala, and Peter Herissone-Kelly, Editors, *Bioethics and Social Reality.* A volume in **Values in Bioethics**